Telling Bodies
Performing Birth

Popular Cultures, Everyday Lives

ROBIN D. G. KELLEY AND JANICE RADWAY, EDITORS

Telling Bodies
Performing Birth

everyday narratives of childbirth

Della Pollock

Columbia University Press

NEW YORK

Columbia University Press
PUBLISHER SINCE 1893
New York   Chichester, West Sussex

Earlier versions of the introduction and chapter one were published in "Origins of Absence: Performing Birth Stories," *TDR: The Drama Review; a journal of performance studies* 41:1 (Spring 1997): 11–42. Reprinted by permission
Excerpts from Eavan Boland, "The Oral Tradition," *Outside History: Selected Poems, 1980–1990* (New York: Norton, 1990) reprinted by permisison of the author.

Library of Congress Cataloging-in-Publication Data
Pollock, Della.
Telling bodies performing birth: everyday narratives of childbirth / Della Pollock.
p. cm. — (Popular culture, everyday lives) Introd. and ch. 1 published in *TDR, the drama review*, 41:1 (Spring 1997).
Includes bibliographical references (p.   ) and index.
ISBN 0–231–10914–8 — ISBN 0–231–10915–6 (pbk.)
1. Women—United States—Social life and customs. 2. Women—United States Interviews. 3. Mothers—United States—Social life and customs. 4. Mothers—United States Interviews. 5. Childbirth—Social aspects—United States. I. Title. II. Series.
HQ1421.P65   1999   98–51186
306.874'3—DC21   CIP

Designed by Ben Farber

Casebound editions of Columbia University Press books are printed on permanent and durable acid-free paper.

Printed in the United States of America
c 10 9 8 7 6 5 4 3 2 1
p 10 9 8 7 6 5 4 3 2 1

For Alan

CONTENTS

ACKNOWLEDGMENTS

Two women
were standing in shadow,
one with her back turned.
Their talk was a gesture,
an outstretched hand.

They talked to each other,
and words like "summer,"
"birth," "great-grandmother"
kept pleading with me,
urging me to follow.

I HAVE TO BEGIN AT THE BEGINNING, with warmest thanks to those people with whom this book is perhaps most deeply entwined, whose collaboration marks every page, into whose arms I left my babies and little kids, whose hard work I cannot match, and who gave me an abiding vision of what it can mean to care. I am forever indebted to Kathy Black, Susan Mansbach, Melanie Pipes, Alison Robertson, Carey Sharpe, and all of the teachers at the Carolina Friends Chapel Hill Early School.

Long before this book began, there was Grace Paley, whom I've read and only met: thanks especially for Faith and "other mothers."

To all the people who gave so much time and energy to the interviews on which this book is based: for purposes of confidentiality, I cannot name you here but hope against hope that the book is testament to your courage and generosity, and to my deepest gratitude. I have chosen to focus on only a few of the interviews in order to provide for more intensive discussion and representation. My sincerest apologies to those of you whose words appear in spirit and shadow only, if not actually in print.

This is a densely social document. I can't tell you how many times just mentioning it has licensed comparisons, correctives, and more and more stories, all of which assured me in every way, every time, that I hadn't said enough, could never say enough, and had, as often as I'd made one point, missed another. It takes no false modesty to say that I loved every time someone told me I was flat out wrong or ran over my end of the conversation with their own; it has taught me, again and again, the limits of explanation—and that this book can, thankfully, always only be a preface to more of the same.

In these sometimes suddenly raw conversations, I was repeatedly moved to think that the power and pleasures of *telling performing* birth were way beyond my or any one person's control. I have often felt, perhaps most important, that working on this project—even as working on it has coursed through births and deaths, trauma and unspeakable joy in my own life—has been what must be an ongoing lesson in, as one woman described her response to an extraordinarily long pregnancy, "surrendering . . . to being out of control." This certainly has its ups and downs. I am grateful to so many people's words, stories, images, looks, laughter, and help for making me believe that's good.

For a start, I'd like to thank Peter Amster, Patrick Anderson, Michael Bowman, Ruth Bowman, Deborah Breen, Amy Ruth Buchanan, Gretchen Case, Barbara Claypole-White, Dwight Conquergood, Jane Danielewicz, Elaine Deerwater, Erik Doxtader, Erica Eisdorfer, Judith Farquhar, Leah Florence, Frank Galati, Kelly Gallagher, Esther Glaser, Beth Grabowski, Lawrence Grossberg, Rachel Hall, Jane Harwell, Mary Frances HopKins, Jodi Kanter, Susan Klebanow, Shannon Jackson, Laurie Lathem, Beverly Whitaker Long, John McGowan, D. Soyini Madison, Michele Mason, Mark Olson, Kevin Parker, Ippy Patterson, Eric E. Peterson, Peggy Phelan, Erica Rothman, Sara Schneckloth, Lori Schneider, Elin O'Hara Slavick, Sara Snow, Mary Susan Strine, James Thompson, Susan Wilson, the anonymous reviewers whose comments enormously improved the manuscript, and the students in courses on performance and oral history, performance and sexuality/visuality, and performance and cultural studies who pressed me (directly and indirectly) to think with them about this work.

Posthumous homage to Dr. Roland Rude, who first gave me performance.

At Columbia University Press: many thanks to my editor, Ann Miller, for imagining this with me in the first place and for providing, in equally large and necessary amounts, patience and push; her assistant, Alex Thorp; Susan Pensak, for assiduous (and encouraging) editing; and to Jan Radway and Robin D. G. Kelley for the privilege of being part of this series.

And then there are those people who just made things possible, who read more than anyone should ever have to, and who I'll always feel honored to call members of my writing group: Jane Blocker, Jacquelyn Dowd Hall, Joy Kasson, and Carol Mavor. Where I have failed to take their wise advice, I accept all responsibility.

Finally, simply, thanks to my parents, Betty and Earl Pollock, for birth, family, and endless devotion; to Nat and Isabel, for life; to Alan, for love and beauty above all.

This book was supported by grants from the Special Projects Fund of the National Communication Association and the University Research Council at the University of North Carolina at Chapel Hill, and by research leaves provided by the Institute for the Arts and Humanities and the College of Arts and Sciences at the University of North Carolina (special thanks to Ruel Tyson and V. William Balthrop for these). Draft versions of chapters 1 and 2 were presented at annual meetings of the International Communication Association (1997), the Association for Theatre in Higher Education (1996), and the PSI/Performance Studies Conference (1996).

One moment I was standing
not seeing out,
only half-listening

staring at the night; the next
without warning
I was caught by it:
the bruised summer light,
the musical subtext

of mauve eaves on lilac
and the laburnum past
and shadows where the lime
tree dropped its bracts
in frills of contrast

where she lay down
in vetch and linen
and lifted up her son
to the archive
they would shelter in . . .
FROM EAVAN BOLAND, "THE ORAL TRADITION"

Telling Bodies
Performing Birth

BIRTH STORIES ARE EVERYWHERE AND NOWHERE. Seen in every movie theater but heard only in brief gasps of attention in grocery store lines or parking lots, inculcated in prenatal classrooms but shamed to the edges of conversation, birth stories permeate and haunt our everyday lives. All too much here and barely there, birth stories embody in miniature long and wide histories of sometimes violent knowledge practices. They (re)produce maternal subjects. They rehearse the body politics at the heart of debates over reproductive technologies, genetic engineering, abortion rights, welfare reform, and custody law, signifying a contest for control over the meaning and value of giving birth of which they are, in turn, a vital part.

For many years now I have been more and less intentionally listening to birth stories. In line, in the hall, over coffee, at the park, and in informal interview settings I have participated in the ritual process of recounting birth "experiences" or, rather, of constituting those experiences out of the scraps of memory and bits of stories left after the ritual performance of birth itself.[1] I heard my first birth story near the end of my first pregnancy—when my round belly and hips betrayed the fact that I would soon be the subject of similar stories, that I was, for all intents and purposes, whether I liked it or not, already inside this particular narrative ring. Bound by a conspiracy of the body, contracted by maternity to hear, to tell, and to retell what others—insidiously, joyously, anxiously—told and retold me, I became both the subject *of* and subject *to* birth stories. Listening, I was the naive student, the initiate, the mother, the co-mother, the sister and friend; I was the bearer of stories; the professional (allied by doing research to institutions of medicine and science), the expert, the surveyor of "good" and "bad" births, the teacher, the outsider who should know or know better.

The first story I heard left me devastated and hungry for more. I was living in a small patrician town outside of Boston at the time (we'd arrived three months earlier and would leave again in two) and was fully nine months pregnant. I'd taken to wandering the streets in the late afternoon, enjoying the sudden, knowing smiles, the uncharacteristic deference of Boston drivers waiting patiently for me to cross the street, the general sense of surrounding pause. I was an intimate stranger to this town. My neighbors—the people I didn't know and would never know who nonetheless used the same dry cleaners and waited at the same stoplights—tended me with fascination. They traded benevolence for participation. As I later learned was so common, they felt the uncommon suspense of an imminent birth and wanted to be in on the drama, conventionally asking, "When are you due?" often reaching out to touch the belly that seemed to reach out to them. I always backed away from these gestures, resisting seduction into mere public property. I wanted to reserve my body's secrecy, to assert my proprietary rights, to protect the zone of privacy with which I had once shielded myself and that now seemed to be so quickly slipping away.

In retrospect I was smug about my ability to walk what seemed a fine but clear line between public and private worlds. I lost my perfect balance one day in the neighborhood grocery. As I wended my way toward the produce section, I admired a young infant sitting straight up in the seat of a grocery cart. Her mother was trying to negotiate the cart, an anxious two- or three-year-old boy, and the last of the summer squash. We exchanged a few pleasantries. Then I was captive. With no warning and heedless of all conventional concerns (including the line forming at our backs and the fact that her son had disappeared down the cereal aisle), she launched into a horrific tale of labor and delivery. Gesticulating wildly over the cabbages and cucumbers, she punctuated her story with frequent, repeated declarations of its main points—"It was a nightmare" and "I will never have another child"—and demonstrated exactly where the emerging fetus had broken through the vaginal wall to the bowel. I don't remember many other details of her story. What I do remember—vividly, so vividly that even now my heart races at the thought—was the dramatic urgency with which she told it and my own flight (such as it was) to the place that was and wasn't my home (now more and less than ever) to retell it to my husband and to whomever else would listen.

This stranger's strange story became part of my body, my experience. It left me shuddering at the proximity of the birth canal and bowel—a closeness I'd simply never dared to consider. Nor had I ever considered, much less felt, that the expansion of one might rip open the other, that each tunnel might not only contract and stretch wildly but spill, break into the other, leaving the body's excremental and reproductive functions separated by only the sheerest strip of torn skin. The woman in the grocery store was clearly still tortured by this indistinction—physically, imaginatively, morally. And, as I listened to her, I accepted the burden of this unimagined and unimaginable experience and, with it, the possibility of a new kind of pleasure, a pleasure drawing me toward a place unkempt with desire, shorn of social convention, constrained only by a deeper, tacit contract that stipulated she would tell and I would listen—and bear her story to others.

Indeed, this was my first birth. It was a rupture in the crafted serenity of my daily life, a breach that induced the anguish and transport of birth liminalities, that defined subsequent incessant performances of self and story, and that required accommodation. I found myself (beyond myself) at once taming and containing the impact of this story through the accumulation and comparison of other stories and renewing its novelty, turning again, by telling it again and again, to the origins of life-in-story. An immeasurable displacement, this was also a threshold experience: it was an initiation into terror mitigated by awe. I was dumbstruck. Other people *knew* this—what she knew, what I now knew: the terror and the secret. I had stumbled into a secret society to which, it seemed, I already belonged. I belonged to her, then as I do now in memory. Whatever solicitude or taboo might have kept us apart now drew us together, confounding the distance between strangers, between memory and forgetting, between the image of that pink-and-bows baby (I could almost smell her sweet warmth; I wanted to cup her strong shoulders and back in my would-be mother's hand) and her mother's ravaged body, between the mother's story and the fact that she was telling it in the *produce* section, for God's sake, between my practiced ideal birth and the frailty of those body walls on which it was so precariously perched. The story put all our carefully plotted means of controlling our (shameful) bodies to shame. Armed with its power, trembling under its threat, I entered into community with women who knew what it meant to be profaned by one's own body, something I was in fact yet to learn and yet knew now more certainly than I ever had or would.

Most of the stories I heard after this one, however, were essentially comic. While only a few closed with complete satisfaction, most rose out of even the depths of terror and anger to embrace the emerging baby and the norms by which it was deemed healthy and whole. Whatever critique a story offered, it was more often than not tempered by expressions of gratitude to the institutions that protected the mother and/or child's health. Most stories followed the linear, "progressive" structure inculcated in prenatal classes and pregnancy handbooks by which planning becomes conception becomes pregnancy becomes a ten-fingers-and-toes birth—the "nine months and counting" model of birth storytelling. Several even seemed licensed by what medical discourses designate a "good outcome" to elaborate and to embellish the preceding dangers and conflict, with the effect, whether intentional or incidental, of improving the climax, of ensuring relief in the final orderliness of all things. With all the flourish of a Shakespearean comedy, they delivered order from disorder and pleasure from abandon, transgression, and pain.

A friend called this the "almost-but" structure of birth stories—stories that torture his memory of his first daughter's stillbirth not with their happiness per se but with the extent to which the expression of that happiness depends on what he called "flirting" with death: exposing the possibility of death or deformity only to deny it. These stories and the performances of these stories offer us a peephole onto the hazy presence of danger. They play with disaster, knowing it will be cast out or contained within the comic structure of the story. They tease us into a kind of freak-show confidence in our own normality and, in turn, invite a sense of superiority to death, disaster, and deformity, as if all it takes to avoid such ends is the proper exercise of courage and technology, as if death were a moral failure and abnormality were the cost of betraying the social order.

Hence it has become common practice in prenatal classes to pass what seem the most benign of the doctor's emergency instruments—forceps, suction, the screw end of the internal fetal monitor—hand to hand, lap to lap, around the room. Met sometimes with a gentle stroke, sometimes a nervous giggle or disgusted grunt, these are sex toys turned inside out. They invite our imaginations to play over their smooth surfaces, to feel their promise, and to anticipate their urgent use. Their very sterility—now marred by touch and fingerprints—suggests the trace of pubic hair and bone, a bleeding perineum, a vaginal canal plugged by a thick and tender fetal scalp. As they move from one expectant parent to the next, marking the ritual circle, they seem to gather totemic force. The more they are touched, tried, rubbed, discarded, the more they seem capable of warding off the very disaster they invoke.

Even the accompanying bubbly chat—"When are you due?" "Boy or girl?"—secures expectations for a happy end. Ritually repeated, reiterated, cited, it locks new parents into a narrative script that simply lacks room for stillbirth, miscarriage, abortion, all deformity—aberrations in the "normal" scheme of things apparently too embarrassing or too grotesque to mention. While the taboos against talking about birth are beginning to erode (I recently heard a cashier at a local hardware store regale an attentive customer with his daughter's birth experience, detail for detail, push for push), they remain strong—and seem even to be getting stronger—against talking about so-called failed births. What talk there is (of "bad" outcomes and absent lives) seems a cursory, obligatory, brief, and uncomfortable break from the routine silence, a kind of toll paid to all the friends and family members waiting for the *news*.

One woman with whom I spoke reported how a friend of hers had called to announce a stillbirth. "I have something unpleasant to tell you," the caller began—as if she were both guilty of being "unpleasant" and under duress to confess her guilt. A friend related a recent miscarriage in short fits and starts, nervously laughing, hot, sweaty, finally noting how the hospital staff had even eliminated the language of "miscarriage" from her medical history, graphing it into her chart (which she was reprimanded for reading) as a "therapeutic abortion"—suggesting to Nina that she should feel both responsible for the termination of her pregnancy (having in effect had an "abortion") and indebted to the medical staff for "therapeutically" redeeming her from the attending guilt.[2] Stories with dire conclusions are often simply prohibited, either by doctors who warn prospective mothers off anecdotes and lore for fear of panic or noncompliance or by the generations of mothers who think they're doing newcomers a favor by not revealing the "secret." Another friend related how comforted she had been by a labor nurse's story of living through her infant's congenital illness and death at six months. The nurse was fired soon after, apparently for sharing this story with other women whose bodies and lives similarly ached with the possibility of telling this story themselves.

In the face of such a forced and awkward silence, death seems both more mysterious and more impossible, both more monstrous for not being seen and more tractable, less frightening, for appearing only as the dragon slain. Death is what medicine overcomes. It is the antagonist vanquished in a morality play acted out over and over again in birth stories. Should death occur, the deep story goes, it must be by some fault of the mother— some failure to comply with medical exigencies or some congenital weakness that makes her shamefully immune to medical help. She must have been rebellious or unsuited from the outset, the silence seems to say. The advantages of hearing how a mother survived her loss or how the medical system let *her* down—rather than she it—disappear in the wake of such a silence. As Michel de Certeau has observed, death is "the unnameable" not because we lack words for it but because the language of the flesh, the "lexicon of the mortal," in which we speak and experience birth, death, and their many strange intersections is an embarrassment to discourses of scientific progress (de Certeau 1984:198).

To the extent that the birth stories that are told and heard are comic-heroic, to the extent that their example further shames stories of death and deformity into silence, they may be complicitous with the system they often otherwise reject: they may convey the same threats and promises that finally moved at least one of the mothers I talked with to concede that a C-section she had vigorously opposed "could've been good." Directly and indirectly, they may support the norms—the desires and expectations for a "normal" birth—enforced by medical practice.

Of course, my husband says (continuing the conversation begun that fateful day at Wellesley). Of course, no one wants to lose a baby, no one wants a child to suffer. We all feel hostage to fortune at times of birth and cling to whatever fragile provisional bits of hope we can find. This is not just social policing, he remonstrates with some indignation, and then reminds me of his own obsession with the possibility that our son might be born with a harelip. I laugh, remembering how he had tamed all his worries to this relatively minor complaint, how he had looked for and found its foreshadows everywhere (suddenly the newspaper seemed full of stories about harelip surgeries and treatments). Of course, I return, but what warrants such worry? What does it say about us that the least variation must be prevented, corrected, or hidden away? And what about those differences that won't yield to the surgeon's gloved hand and scalpel, differences that remain "spectacularly visible" like sex and skin color or that are invisible at the outset, closeted away in an apparently healthy body, awaiting performance, like mental disability or sexual preference (Barker 1984:24)? In the rush of our "natural" desire to guard against the whimsy and ravages of nature, do we naturalize social disdain for difference? To what extent, in our fear of pathology, do we pathologize—and create the very suffering we want to avoid?

In the next chapter I will focus on stories that challenge the comic-heroic norm of birth storytelling with news of its failures and injustices. I will consider stories that take their pulse from a gap, a breach in the system, an absence wrought by pressure either to keep death quiet or to meet heterosexual, marital, and medical norms. These stories follow from silence or a marked *difference*. They call the outside of conventional birth stories *in*, making silence echo through birth storytelling, challenging the power of conventional genres to keep death and difference out, recalling the power of performance not only to create something from nothing, or even nothing from something, but to re-present nothing at all—to yield presence to absence in the troubled and troubling act of reckoning with what's not known or unknown, or with what may be unknowable.[3]

These stories, like those addressed in subsequent chapters, resist shame and silence, at least in part, by throwing off narrative norms. When I asked my mother about my own birth, she tried to accommodate my interest. Over sour pickles and chicken soup she began with the crazy car chase to the hospital, paused, stumbled, "And there you were!" Her story, like what we typically think of as a good story, had a beginning and end—but no middle. She was "knocked out" for the delivery, eager but able only to construct a story out of conventional narrative tropes ("Going to the hospital") and the logic of efficiency/outcomes. What loomed in the middle silence was the unspoken because unquestioned authority of medical science.

What became painfully clear throughout the interviews for this project, and the conversations that trailed through and around its every aspect, was that "birth stories" are not limited to accounts of labor and delivery. Their center shifts with each telling. Given the opportunity, women made what is typically left to the margins of birth discourse—the mother's body, prenatal deaths, sex, conception, genetic counseling—the primary subjects of their birth stories. In so doing, they achieved alternative, if ragged and fleeting, forms of subjectivity: they claimed affective authority; they reclaimed rights to maternal identity; they threw open doors dividing death and birth, sex and birth, sex and death to carnival indistinction. As the subjects of their own stories, they became who they were in narrative performance. They became themselves *becoming* . . . subjects, narrators, actors, given, possible, impossible, and intolerable selves. They subjected themselves, and me, and you, to often unnerving, transforming articulations of memory, discourse, and desire.

This book is about maternal subjects—about the things women (and men) talk about when they talk about birth and about the selves that emerge when they talk about those things. It is, in the end, about talking understood as performance—as the artful, inventive, changing, interstitial, corporeal process of negotiating the meaning and value of birth and as the means by which the narrating self authorizes new selves, alliances, and norms of relation, even as she reveals the deep impress of norms and expectations on herself.

Understood as performance, birth stories dramatize the convergence of multiple stories on the birth experience. They undermine the presumed neutrality of medical procedures and the apparent transparency of birth experiences with the pressure of their own reflexivity, effectively hot-wiring a network of rituals and resistances composed at least in part of medical technodramas, religious and secular rites (baptisms, baby showers), prenatal pedagogies, media fantasies (Murphy Brown singing "You make me feel like a natural woman" to her baby boy, just minutes after giving birth on prime-time TV, Hugh Grant finding celebrity redemption in *Nine Months*, Xena the Warrior Princess performing a cesarean section on the Amazon mother of a centaur-baby boy, hypothetical, sci-fi horrors reported in *Glamour* magazine, Demi Moore, naked *and* pregnant on the cover of *Vanity Fair*), toy-play that makes adoption seem as easy as buying a Cabbage Patch baby and birth as neat and easy as substituting the flat for the round abdominal panel on the new "Mommy-To-Be"-cum-Barbie doll, dirty jokes, body styles, compulsive performances of the "good mother," subaltern raids on official birth discourses, and the birth narratives that, in various forms, pervade, mock, and sustain all of the above.

Looping through multiple performativities, birth stories threaten not only the conventional isolation of birth from other episodes in the formation of cultural identity but also the concomitant isolation of birth from the broader body politics of, for instance, abortion, sexual orientation, reproductive technologies, "family values," welfare and healthcare reform. Birth stories put the maternal body—in all its carnal, social, and political plenitude—center stage. They counter puritanical, masculinist, racist, classist, and even feminist bans on the birthing body with its embodied representation, doubling the threat of female embodiment to the norms of a phallogocentric culture.[4]

In the second and third chapters I consider birth story performances as counterrites and practices—as re/ritualizations of maternal identity and as discursive strategies in a contest over pain. Chapter 2, "Narrative Rites," focuses on one narrative encounter that was in fact a four-part improvisation on recent developments in reproductive technology—a bluesy, brazen replay of its main themes and formulae, especially insofar as they construct and confer "fertility."

Chapter 3, "Practicing Pain," challenges the common assumption that pain is prelinguistic. In the light of wildly divergent, lyrically cogent, and sometimes painfully critical birth stories, it argues that vernacular discourses practice pain *differently*: they refuse the dereliction of birth pain (often referred to as "discomfort" by medical staff and handbooks) to neurology and hysteria, performing instead—in metaphor, image, laughter, and grief—a wide-ranging logics and politics of pain that exceed scientific normativities and masculinist discourses that insist on the prerational, asyntactical nature of pain—with which the maternal body is typically identified. In part or whole, as one among many: birth stories unname pain or name it differently. They are a form of discursive practice that, heard and felt, defies the Cartesian denial of body knowing and blast open its concomitant categories of gender, sex, meaning, and value.

In chapter 4, "Secrets/Doubles," I suggest that some birth stories depend on silence or some measure of secrecy for their effectiveness. They appropriate silence for their own ends: Charlotte revels in what amounts to secret witness to her "accidental" homebirth; Ruth rehearses the way she blinkered the hospital system, slipping in and out of a race and class-based bureaucracy; Ellen parses her story in careful detail, revealing most pointedly what she concealed—the underground protocols of home-birthing in a state that bans lay midwifery—performing *secrecy*, reciting the power of *in*visibility for her own ends.

Even, or perhaps especially, in the half-silences of whispered, abrupt, withheld performances, birth stories articulate the intersection of other stories, other performances: stories of the birthing body, the body as story, embodied stories. Birth stories are always already performed. And yet their danger consists in their originality: in their origins in performance and in their power to establish origins. As performances, they are unique constructions of bodies in space-time. They disappear into subsequent, often discontinuous reckonings and performances, challenging preferences for more linear abstract modes of knowledge formation with their immediacy, contingency, and particularity.[5] As minor myths of origin, moreover, they loan history (however narrowly or broadly defined) the authority of beginnings; through repetition and condensation, they become the founding "facts" of history, the origin and ground from which history derives its sense of purpose. In other words, the originality of birth stories consists in centering history in the convergences of performativity and maternity: in making history subject to the maternal body performing itself in ritual, spectacle, and story and in trading on the slippery promise of performative origins.

Birth stories consequently imply a radical inversion of established structures of meaning and action and so must be, it seems, counterperformed. They must be circumscribed, discredited, pushed to the margins of discursive practice, whether by pejorative identification with "gossip," "lore," and "anecdote" or by the use of anesthetics that either remove the birthing woman from her body, and her body from its story, or make her body—and so her story—conform to prescribed medical narratives or by social protocols that license the carnival play of birth storytelling for "a few days" or "two weeks" or possibly a year after a child's birth only to secure its subsequent submission to codes of privacy, decency, and domesticity. Accordingly, a friend and mother of three grown boys asked of this project, "What is there to tell?"

Listening again and again to the many stories I heard through the course of this project (on tape, in dreams, even as I retell them and tell them again here), I want to recover their disappearance in time (to which they are, as performances, productively disposed) from their disappearance in discourse (to which they are, as performances, condemned). I want to perform their implications for history: to pursue their likely sedimentations, to mine their ambivalences and contradictions, to widen the gaps charged, the differences wrought, with each recurrence. I want to renew their respective attempts to gain at least symbolic dominion over the birthing process and, in the spirit of our "original" conversations, to keep their meanings in play—to underwrite their ongoing performativity with my own reflections on the ways in which each simultaneously counters and constitutes social, sexual, and scientific norms. In so doing I hope to write the possibilities of a maternal performativity into performance and cultural studies but, more important, to supplement those studies with the pleasures and power of telling birth.

****

The stories told throughout this book are about giving birth from the mid-eighties to the mid-nineties in and around Chicago and Boston, and in the southeast region of the United States. But, as stories about contemporary birthing, they refer to a long history that is as often apparent in its marked absence—in remarks about what these mothers' mothers didn't or wouldn't tell them (either because the common use of general anesthesia in the fifties and early sixties left few memories to tell or because generational social codes made such talk inappropriate, bad, embarrassing, taboo) as it is in detours through the recent past to grandmothers' tales. It was not uncommon for the women I talked with to skip back a generation to a time when homebirthing was still routine and doctors and hospitals were for the dead and dying. One woman, anticipating a homebirth, recalled her grandmother's concern about who was going to make her "tick" ("The thing they made that had layers of newspaper and then muslin and you sewed it together in a quilted way and it's where you birthed your baby"). Another recounted how matter of factly her grandmother had carried the body of a stillborn baby to the hospital for final disposition before burial. Another reveled in the way her grandmother, privileged by enduring faith and coded reticence about female sexuality (two women that had lived together for years were understood to be "very good friends"), embraced her granddaughter's lesbian relationship.

This is a history of increasingly centralized medical practice, or what is commonly called "medicalization": the process by which medical and technical expertise overtook not only both ends of life, birth and death, but changed the way we understand our bodies, making them objects of abstract, anatomical knowledge systems, largely unintelligible except by clinical translation.[6] The birth stories recounted in this book operate in and against the silences produced by medicalization—they claim the discourses deferred along chains of prenatal testing, cut off by anesthesia, made to conform to textbook models, or suppressed within matrices of normative masculinity and heterosexuality.[7]

With the rise of the hospital in the early twentieth century, bodily life was disentangled from the social rites and economies in which it was traditionally enmeshed. Birthing, like dying, was removed from domestic public spaces.[8] Domestic spaces, in turn, ceased to be public. By the fifties the lines dividing public and private spaces were sharply drawn, not only delimiting women's role in a postwar economy but isolating women from each other, making them subject instead to the idealization of the white middle-class family popularized by TV shows and advertising and to the authority of (male) medical practitioners.

As Judith Leavitt shows in her remarkable study, *Brought to Bed: Childbearing in America, 1750–1950*, medical control over birth literally corresponds to the change in birthplace. Although by the turn of the twentieth century women conventionally invited male doctors to attend deliveries and availed themselves of a variety of medical, technical interventions, birth remained a woman-centered practice. Set in a domestic scene flush with relatives and neighbors, women retained authority over birth. Their consolidated social power meant that birth was women's lot and terrain. As Leavitt explains:

> The psychologically vital presence of trusted women friends, despite the influence of male medicine, continued to shape much of the childbirth experience for individual women. Men could be asked to do some things, restrained from doing others; they could be argued with and agreed with; but rarely were they allowed to make decisions on their own. Thus medicine changed the birth experience, but only within the limits set by women's birthing-room culture. The gender-based context in which women gave birth continued in this country until birth moved to the hospital, until it physically was no longer part of women's world. (LEAVITT 1986:203)

Nineteenth-century urbanization and mobility took its toll on women's social networks. By the turn of the century it left many women stranded, without the convenience of nearby friends and relatives. At the same time, the new sciences promised reduced maternal and infant mortality. Enlightenment rhetoric made the hospital seem not only a practical but a necessary alternative to the more ad hoc environment of the homebirth. The hospital, by the mid-twentieth century, began to redeem its promise of safer births.

And yet the ideal of a safe birth had its costs, among them the collapse of women's birthing culture and the power that culture secured for women as women. The hospital birth removed the birthing woman from the gender- and often faith-based context of homebirth as well as from the web of everyday social, symbolic relations in which homebirth thrived. It sacrificed the rich social history that brought women together in the birthing room—often across family and community lines—to the efficiency and sterility of the hospital ward. Routinely isolated, drugged, and often physically restrained, the woman giving birth in a hospital in the early part of the twentieth century was literally cut off from all social resources. She was not only physically but socially debilitated. As a result, her agency was easily usurped by the attending physician. Indeed, by the 1920s, "Women were no longer the main actors; instead, physicians acted upon women's bodies" (Leavitt 1986:190). Without the provisions of a women's culture—social solidarity, empathy, traditional wisdom, shared values, manual skills, domestic help and, above all, a common sense of the importance and difficulty of birthing and mothering—the birthing woman lost control over both her experience and the means of interpreting it. Deprived of its determinations within women's culture, birth became less a sign of women's power than a symbolic internment of female passivity.

The homebirth of the late nineteenth century was not, however, uncontested. It was, rather, a gendered battleground over which women generally prevailed. With the rise of hospital obstetrics, women eventually surrendered their advantage. The largely male obstetric profession dismissed women's reluctance to go to the hospital as trivial next to its assurance of safety, arguing that the fact that " 'women love their homes and abhor the idea of going to the hospital for the purpose of confinement is only a sentiment begotten of custom and deserves no special refutation. Let women once appreciate that the hospital is the safest place for them to pass through the ordeal of labor, they will seek it of their own accord.' "[9]

And women did seek it of their own accord. Hospital birthing was not a conspiracy wrought by men against women. It had specific, sometimes insidious, implications for gender relations, pitting as it did "home," "sentiment," and "custom" against rationalized, specialized birth management. It broke the connections between birth and social life that had imbued the act of giving birth with social power. It weakened longstanding traditions of domestic control and alliance that had sustained at least bipartite worlds of production and reproduction. And it neutralized birth by atomizing it, by compartmentalizing it as a routine procedural incident, separate from the complex politics of everyday living.

But the history of birthing in the United States is part of the larger history of industrialization, a history driven by general confidence in the advantages of scientific and technological "progress." Men and women shared this vision. Both were driven—although perhaps for different reasons—to perfect the birth process. Both were deeply invested in what has been generally characterized as a "masculine" ideology of control over the body as a material object: a machine, literally a means of production. Indeed the rise in reproductive technologies—from the use of anesthesia and forceps to cesarean section, in vitro fertilization, and surrogacy—has been fueled by a middle class eager not only to maintain lines of biological descendance and inheritance but to exercise its rights and power to purchase within what would become an industrial economy of (re)production.[10]

The exercise of consumer power around birth has had consistently contrary effects. From the outset, it encouraged intervention for its own sake. What distinguished the seventeenth-century *accoucheur* from traditional midwives (besides a lack of experiential knowledge) was his tools—forceps, hooks, and drugs—and he was paid to use them. Despite new awareness of the dangers of bacterial contagion in the nineteenth century (after two centuries of puerperal fever), antisepsis remained weak and interventionist practice remained crude, mechanical, and intrinsically dangerous. The common result was increased infection and worse complications. The irony of the situation was not lost on one physician who explained: " 'Perhaps the best way to manage normal labor is to let it alone, but you cannot hold down a job and do that.' "[11] The obstetrician (even in his early incarnations as male midwife and barber-surgeon) relied on women for his livelihood and women relied on the talismanic charm of medical instruments. Within the emergent matrix of production and consumption, doctors and mothers participated together in the denial and denigration of traditional midwives.[12] By the early part of the twentieth century the doctor with the greatest number of tools was the most prestigious, the most sought after, and the best paid.

Nowhere is the irony of woman's role as the consumer of medical novelties more evident than in the history of "twilight sleep." After the publication of an article in *McClure's Magazine* in 1914 describing a new method of painless childbirth that had gained popularity in Germany, women's and feminist organizations in the United States rallied together to demand the use of scopolomine-morphine in childbirth. While American doctors remained wary of its effects on both mother and infant and were initially reluctant to provide the specialized care it required, women saw "scope" as an end to the fear and suffering of birth. They moreover saw it as a cause celebre, a vehicle for recovering the right to control the birth environment. Paradoxically, under the influence of scope, birthing mothers entered into a half-conscious state: their minds were completely shut off from the activity of their bodies—which remained vigorous, even wild and violent. They yielded control over the birth per se to the physicians who protected their patients by keeping them in crib-beds or bed-cages (hospital beds specially fitted with sheeted sides and top). Relieved of the pain associated with birth, scoped-out women were also relieved of the memory of birth. They were increasingly alienated from their bodies and personal maternal histories. Set adrift from themselves, it is not hard to imagine that women were subsequently more afraid of giving birth and more susceptible to the appeal of anesthesia. In effect, women subsidized proof that they were weak, "nervous," and—like the children or wild animals they became in "twilight sleep"—needed paternalistic restraint. Their demands for scope and anesthesia more generally thus supported the rise of obstetric specialization and the consolidation of hospital-run birthing practices.[13]

The natural childbirth movement of the sixties and seventies challenged the effects of medicalization on gender identification through the formation of homebirthing cooperatives, the compensations of "spiritual midwifery," and increased pressure on doctors to attend "awake and aware" births. While it was not uncommon for a woman to be "knocked out" as soon as she arrived at the hospital, whether she was experiencing early contractions or (as one woman reported) the baby was already crowning, women were now cautioned against coming to the hospital too soon or they would be "sent home." In living rooms and local Ys, they trained in the masculinist, mind-over-matter methods spearheaded by Fernand Lamaze and Grantly Dick-Read (and taken to a new height in the "Bradley method") that were no more or less "natural" than either medicated births or births embedded in the history and culture of homebirthing. Still paternalistic in its orientation (epitomized in the title of the popular book, *Thank You, Dr. Lamaze*), the Lamaze method emphasized arcane breathing techniques timed to regulated birth phases. It was quickly absorbed into the new form of hospital-based "prepared childbirth" classes—classes devoted to reducing stress and thus both pain and panic by familiarizing students with all the tests and procedures they might encounter in the hospital setting—including genetic testing, ultrasound diagnosis, internal and external monitoring, episiotomy, induction, epidural, and cesarean section. Birth preparation classes provide a primer on the hospital birth. Often sponsored by hospitals or obstetric groups, they enculturate students in scientific and institutional norms. They give anxious parents enough knowledge to feel "in the know," but usually only enough to feel indebted to physician recommendations. In general, they preempt opposition by positioning students *inside* the hospital culture.

Hospital-based prenatal classes left living room (or local Y) Lamaze sessions in their wake (making them seem cartoon quaint). In effect, medical enculturation renewed itself, and its centripetal momentum, in the natural childbirth movement, eliding whatever remained of the domestic with technosphere birthing that allowed for a full range of medical supplements to cut the pain without compromising commitments to being awake and aware. And yet, as Robbie Davis-Floyd has argued, women who are awake and aware are more susceptible to ritual subordination than women who are unconscious (knocked out and unknowing). Davis-Floyd distinguishes between the effects of scopolomine, general anesthesia, and the now common use of epidurals to anesthetize only the lower half of the body:

> To fully understand the symbolic significance of the epidural in hospital birth, we need to consider the meaning of its replacement of scopolamine and general anesthesia as routine procedures in most hospitals. Although "scope" did serve to reinforce the technological model of birth, in that it told women that their machines did not need them to produce a baby, it did not make women act like machines but like wild animals—an uncomfortable metaphor that undermined society's attempts to make birth appear to be mechanical enough to conform to the reality created by the technological model. Furthermore, any type of general anesthesia meant that the woman would miss many of the important messages she could be receiving. The "awake-and-aware" Lamaze patient with the epidural fits the picture of birthing reality painted by the technological model much better than the "scoped out" or "gassed out" mother, for the epidural makes a physical reality out of the conceptual separation of mind and body, a reality that the woman will grasp precisely because of her awareness. (DAVIS-FLOYD 1992:166)

Administered through an IV drip attached to the lower spine, the epidural also leashes the birthing mother to the bed, limiting her range of both motion and thought in a way reminiscent of the scopolamine cages, although, in the case of the epidural, with complete, if not always acute, awareness of her constraints.[14]

The social environment of the hospital birth has also changed. Perhaps one of the most significant and contradictory effects of the natural childbirth movement has been the repositioning of male partners within the hospital culture. Whereas early hospital regimens isolated birthing women not only from other women but from their partners and families, the husband waiting it out by the phones is now basically a relic preserved in sitcoms. Men are generally congratulated on their involvement in the traditionally female terrain of blood and birth. Hailed as "coach" and nonmedical ally, men stand in for the women companions of yesteryear. But this is not an unproblematic substitution. While men's involvement does signal an at least partial recovery of the social context of homebirth, it also marks the privatization of birth within the heterosexual nuclear family. It limits the explicitly social relevance of birth to the legally and conventionally sanctioned relationship between husband and wife. As one of the men I talked with indicated, the birth process has come to be known as "a couples thing." It belongs—in a kind of exclusive and traditionally romantic way—to the lovers who made the baby in the first place. Insofar as the husband-coached birth is something that happens *between* conjugal mates rather than *among* the fluid mix of neighbors and relatives that attended the homebirth, it rehearses the privatization of the modern family. Incorporating men in the birth process opens birth to its social context but closes that context to participants outside the marital unit. It thus enforces prevailing norms of sexuality. (To wit, the tensions that arise around single and lesbian mothers' births as well as in cases where the mother prefers female assistance.) It appears to humanize the birth scene by featuring a primary relationship in the birthing woman's life but accordingly protects the private/public boundaries that delimit the birthing woman's social power.

The husband-coached model may also strengthen men's conventional role within marriage. On the one hand, it diminishes birth by characterizing it as a sport, a competition, over which men exercise a kind of playful authority (often supplemented by "funny" coach T-shirts or even commercial kits complete with "coaching cap, digital stopwatch (to time contractions), sports bottle, counter-pressure ball, hyperventilation bag, time-of-delivery pool card, ear plugs and coaching tips for every phase of labor").[15] On the other hand, it gives men a kind of imperial control they didn't have in the waiting room. It broadens their scope of involvement both *in* and *over* women's lives—such that one woman I talked with (whose story is addressed at length in chapter 3, "Practicing Pain") described her husband as a "savior" and another mourned what amounted to his cruel detachment. Others recounted a deepened sense of closeness and partnership; one simply dismissed her husband as useless; several felt weakened by what seemed their husband's greater, if well-intentioned, allegiance to the medical staff. In all cases, the stories of husband-coached birth suggest that it is an enactment and often an intensification of prior marital relations, relations defined within the larger cultural context of which Lamaze is now a prominent part. In other words, the fact that a man attends his wife's birth is not in and of itself an indication of gender transformation and may actually indicate the opposite: the reinforcement of conventionally paternalistic gender roles. As one interviewee, Karen, put it, the husband-coached model is "not all it's cracked up to be."

Consumer demand is largely responsible for the recent dramatic changes in hospital birthing environments.[16] Today hospitals offer "home-style" birthing rooms, single-room maternity care, such luxury items as jacuzzi showers and whirlpool baths, and even separate birthing centers, recognizing the health value of whole body, whole family care within a competitive market that makes customer satisfaction critical. Among other things, a positive birth experience tends to generate a loyal clientele. Such perqs, however, are often glossier in ads than in reality, are less widespread than the news of them, and—consistent with the profit cycle in which they are produced—may be more show than substance.[17]

These changes are not insignificant. The medical profession has begun to appreciate the fact that multiple interventions may be disabling, that interventions have a domino effect—one necessitates another and so on. A not uncommon scenario runs something like this: the woman who doesn't eat during labor in case of surgery risks nausea, which is treated with drugs that slow labor; she is treated with pitocin, a labor-inducing drug that may make contractions so painful as to require pain killers that at best diminish her direct consciousness of contractions and make her entirely dependent on monitors and medical staff to read her own body. Meanwhile, she has been so immobilized by hunger, IV tubes, monitor straps, and drugs that labor may never regain its original momentum and may require more elaborate and much riskier interventions—from internal fetal monitoring to forceps delivery and cesarean section. The institutional accommodation of more relaxed birthing styles—in the form of birthing rooms and still rare but much celebrated single-room maternity care—reflects awareness that the woman who feels comfortable also feels less pain, requires fewer interventions, and faces fewer complications. But birthing rooms and attending nurse-midwives are also cost-efficient alternatives to delivery rooms and Ob/Gyns. They conveniently serve both the investment interests of the hospital and the psychosocial needs of the birthing mother.

A bit of contemporary birth lore, however, suggests that they may not do so in equal proportion. The common, half-hearted joke among prospective parents and the nursing staff who give the maternity ward tours— "Just move the chintz curtains (or the Renoir print) and there is the monitor (or the oxygen tank or the IV pole)"—indicates ironic critical consciousness of just how deep recent changes go. It betrays a false cheerfulness. It suggests both homes-and-gardens awe at the decorator's sleight of hand ("It doesn't look like a hospital room!") and a wary, quickly repressed concern that whatever's homey here may be only a visual effect.

The tourists usually go on, happily enough, as if in grateful, if rather cynical, agreement that—in this strange but wonderful land—looking like home (or someone's idea of home) will suffice. (It's interesting to note that the spate of singles bars emerging at the same time similarly fetishized the homey, their magazine-perfect living room simulations recalling a lost horizon of something like real intimacy).

Recent consumer movements to demedicalize birth continue to operate, moreover, within contemporary economic and institutional frameworks. They tend to focus narrowly on birth—reflecting the political isolation of birth from other issues of sexuality, reproduction, and gender, including abortion, child care, sexual abuse and harassment—especially insofar as these are layered in discourses of class and race—and the medical isolation of birth even from death. At the same time that they have achieved major concessions to consumer demand, they have also thus contributed to what Adrienne Rich (1986:xii) calls weak, if not backward, reformism:

> To the extent that the alternative-childbirth movement has focused on birth as a single issue, it has been a reform easily subsumed into a new idealism of the family. Its feminist origins have been dimmed along with its potential challenge to the economics and practices of medicalized childbirth and to the separation of motherhood and sexuality.

One aim of this book is to challenge the discourses that encourage us to think about and practice birth in isolation and so, however unwittingly, to serve prevailing body politics. It is meant to reflect the integration of birth and gender, identity, body, sexual, economic, and institutional politics encompassed by birth stories. This book is, in fact, not about birth at all. It is about birth stories. It is about how we use and refashion available narrative forms to articulate pain and "progress," to link birth and its counterpart, sex, and their counterpart, death, to reveal struggles for identity and agency against the micro-, biopolitics of conventional maternities, and to create hidden, alternative, and oppositional body discourses. The book is meant to resist the easy assimilation of birth to the "new idealism of the family" (or what are in fact old family values platforms). I have often been struck by friends' surprise at finding that this book is not "just" about birth or for women as mothers. I have taken heart in their discovery, realizing just how tightly cultural discourses hold even the most sympathetic and sophisticated imaginations, *separating out* birth as the stubborn sign of nature vs. culture, as transparent (feral) experience, as something women do, as the object of specialized medical practices, or as the subject of bioromantic hype (typically favored by anti- and reactionary feminisms that narrowly identify women with their reproductive capacities). And yet, heard in all of their plenitude and excess, birth stories defy the ready isolation of birth. They spill and stain, turning the lines that would otherwise cut them off and keep birth *out* into an inky blur—of which, I hope, this book is one example.

* * * *

All the interviews on which this book is based were informal. Of the thirty-nine men and women interviewed, twenty were members of more and less well-defined groups—a new mothers group, a hospital-based prenatal class, a single mothers support group, and a loose network of married students and their spouses; of those, fourteen were interviewed by established members of the group. The nineteen additional interviewees were friends, friends of friends, and people I didn't know—who had heard about the project and called me. All the women interviewed had had at least one child during the previous five years in the midwest and eastern regions of the United States. I made little or no attempt to secure a scientifically valid sample, in part because I depended on a level of rapport built on prior acquaintance and/or identification, and in part because many of the women and men with whom I spoke sought a nonscientific environment in which to explore, among other things, their relationship to contemporary scientific practices. In this latter regard, there was clearly a politics to my method, although I trust it was one that favored my interviewees' perspectives. With the exception of casual conversations with adoptive parents, all the interviews were with biological parents. Rather than naturalizing maternity, my aim here has been to explore the capacity of the birth narrative to (re)produce the maternal body, to intervene in the politics of the body from the body, assuming that the meanings that circulate around and through women's bodies are contested, shifting, and ambivalent.[18]

The men and women with whom I spoke often seemed caught between the erosion of a coherent, women's birth culture (that no amount of nostalgia can or should restore) and due gratitude to medical protections that have, for the most part, dispelled the "shadow of death" under which preindustrial women birthed. They nonetheless found that the systems on which they relied were not invulnerable. They did not dominate women in any simple or absolute way. They cannot master birth and the birthing woman. To the contrary, the relentlessly unpredictable nature of birth, the body, and pain initiates what must be an ongoing struggle for control over the birth process in which women continue to participate both passively and aggressively.

Women told stories of resisting the alienating effects of the hospital in a variety of ways.[19] Many simply avoided the hospital, either partially or entirely, by delaying going to the hospital or giving birth at home (in one case, elaborated in chapter 4, the former resulted in the latter). They insisted on early discharges. They brought home to the hospital in the form of pictures, pillows, friends. They joked. They used guerrilla tactics and subterfuge—a midwife held her foot against the door to delay the doctor's insistence on a cesarean; one woman gained strength by snacking while the nurses weren't looking. They made sometimes costly trade-offs: two of the women I talked with accepted drugs from a pressing nurse or resident in order to get them off their backs. They engaged in open combat. They followed some prenatal instructors' advice to "go in there and fight"—and risked distraction, enervation, and residual bitterness, not to mention the militarization of their birth experience.

They also pulled against a variety of narrative restraints: a sense of institutional shame, a desire just to forget an experience that often left them bitter and angry, an unwillingness to scare other women, the general isolation of women from other women, whether at work in or out of their homes, a sophisticated distrust of their authority as narrators (typically enforced by parenting magazine columns citing doctors' advice not to listen to other women's anecdotes, old wives' tales, and such word-of-mouth prescriptions for labor induction as spicy food and "castor oil cocktails"), taboos that fence off the body, the personal, and the "impure" from conversation, and a lack of models—with a few notable exceptions, the women with whom I spoke gave birth in the wake of a generational silence: their mothers' births were forgotten to general anesthesia.[20]

They told different kinds and versions of stories (one woman noted, "I should have asked which of the hundred stories you wanted me to tell!"). Some sublimated the experience in symbolic form. Some "confessed" weakness. Many surrogated the act and pleasures of telling for whatever lack or pain they felt in the birth process, confirming Marie Huet's sense that "to retell is to act and thereby claim the pleasure which is deferred in the time of the performance" (Huet 1982:33). With each retelling they echoed and sapped medical, media, and commodity discourses, in each case making the meanings and effects of the birth process a point of public dialogue, refusing to keep birthing, mothering, and family private, closed off, foreclosed. They opened those meanings to collaborative rein-terpretation even as they vigorously directed the dialogue. In general, they struggled to assert symbolic dominion over birth, often in bits and pieces of conversation that looked, for all intents and purposes, like talk about the weather (a woman I'd just met at a pot luck dinner glanced over her shoulder at her mother scolding her daughter and then, with a quick laugh, slid into a description of "that forbidden thing!" her teenage pregnancy, and her daughter's birth: "She just about killed me!"). In scraps torn from others' stories (mothers', doctors', neighbors', tabloid celebrities', TV char-acters') appropriated to their own, they forged unforeseen connections between tellers and listeners and possible listeners, anticipating other per-formances elsewhere, in other spaces between and behind everyday perfor-mances of femininity and mothering.

* * * *

Birth stories migrate. They move in and through history, among tellers and listeners. They are mobile cultural fragments, renewed in affective alliance with other cultural *parts*. They constitute a *partial* culture, a cul-ture that is part this and that, that is deeply invested in its representation-al forays, that is never complete, always in motion, furtive, fugitive, and yet *connected* in something like a diasporic relation of parts—at the vanishing intersection of deliberate and coincidental performances.[21] This book is a *partial* account of a partial performative culture.

It is an intimate ethnography. It is an attempt to write a cultural poli-tics of birth narratives across a wide range of practices and sites in the contemporary United States, drawing on a loose array of new and not so new ethnographic methods—informal oral histories, reflexive cultural cri-tique, identity ethnography, performance anthropology, hearsay, gossip, and personal reflection.[22] It reads/writes instances of cultural praxis, where the embodied body politics of telling birth stories animates, corrects, and exceeds theories of feminist subjectivity, corporeality, popular transgres-sion, and the performance of everyday life.[23]

Part to part, it is an *intimate* account in several senses:

1. I have tried, throughout the book, to evoke the im/mediacies of performance, the moments when one story compels another into being/becoming, where two embodied subjects meet over food, in story, in ges-tures read back and forth, across the borders of bodies, selves, social worlds in the corporeal imaginary of telling birth. I have been inspired, in this

regard, by Trinh Minh-ha's sense of the connection between the erotics and mnemonics of oral transmission.[24] "The words passed down from mouth to ear (one sexual part to another sexual part), womb to womb, body to body," Trinh says, "are the remembered ones" (Trinh 1989:136). Remembering these words, I have listened closely, "body to body," to other people's truths, performing *closeness*, or what Michael Jackson calls an aesthetic and ethic of "being-together-with" (Jackson 1989:8). I have reread these stories through my own memory, body, and imagination, trying at every turn to find what, if anything, was illuminating in my response, what I could return to the story and the reader.

In so doing, I have told a series of *narrative encounters*, each of which has renewed for me Clifford Geertz's early sense that "the growth in range [that] a powerful sensibility gains from an encounter with another one, as powerful or more, comes only at the expense of its inward ease" (Geertz 1983:45). I have tried to account for the claims each encounter made on my "inward ease," knowing that in various ways, to varying extents, each made me uncomfortable, each moved me to ecstasy. I made myself, as much as possible, vulnerable to being moved. Listening and writing, I saw myself as the register of someone else's power. Against the grain of current obsessions with the power of the researcher to shape, tame, appropriate, and control the worlds he or she investigates, in the course of talking with and writing about the many people who contributed to this project, I more often than not felt unnerved and overwhelmed, "othered," interrogated, propelled into landscapes of knowing and not knowing I would not otherwise have dared enter. At the same time, I insisted on the integrity of my own perspectives, my own theoretical and critical sensibilities, without which a dialogue, in the hardest and most meaningful sense of that word, could not have occurred.[25]

2. This is an open book. It is suggestive and rarely conclusive. It is meant to invite the reader into double-play: into performing the book and the stories it conveys *inside out*, participating *in* the conversational dynamics the book replays and taking them *out* again, into a heightened, amplified, expanding alchemy of birth/body stories.[26]

3. It consequently engages what various scholars and critics have called performative writing. I have written elsewhere about what I take to be some of the characteristics and possibilities of performative writing; others have as well, more eloquently than I ever could.[27] As you read this

book, it may be useful to think of it as "performative" in these, among other, ways:

The book lacks a foundational subject.

"I" am featured prominently throughout the book. But I don't take myself—any more than I do any of the other selves that I rehearse—to be the final referent for whatever is said or gained here. What the circuitry of birth storytelling suggests above all is the possibility for staking origins and identities in the "fractal intricacies" of performance (Sedgwick 1993:9), in between the multiple performances that may be encompassed by any one. I traverse performance, following the nerveways that divide and connect identities, communities, ways of knowing and being, tracking "other movements, hopes of becoming, and alternative belongings" (Probyn 1996:14–15).[28] As I suggest in the second chapter, I am "I" because I move; I am the I reworked in processes of enunciation. Speaking, telling, moving inexorably "from her experience to mine, and mine to hers," reconstituting each in turn, I am becoming-other (Probyn 1993:4).

The reflexive *I* in the book is meant to stand in for this performative self, to enact the possibilities of becoming in and through performative relays. It is meant as well to evoke a dialogical relation that, as Allen Feldman argues, "does not require the physical presence of the other; rather, it is all the more powerful in the literal absence of the other, who is present as a violent material and historical effect on language, meaning, and theory" (Feldman 1991:12). To the extent that "I" am I here, I take myself to be the mediated and mediating sign of that effect.

I consequently speak in several languages at once; my tongue is "forked." The language of the book, like the worlds it speaks, is "heteroglot" (Bakhtin 1981:293); it is high, low, mobile, emotional, scenic, descriptive, implicated, inductive, desiring, strategic, mine, not-mine.

The book emphasizes the specificity of stories, selves, and situations.

I have not tried to write a grand taxonomy of birth stories. I do not take any of the stories or selves represented here to be generally "representative." I have resisted throughout the impulse to classify and categorize, to name story genres and types. I have backed off even from drawing comparisons too tightly. Insisting on the relative specificity of each story and situation, I have tried to avoid reiterating the normalizing models of scientific discourse with which most of the women with whom I spoke struggled. I have also tried to sustain the singularity of each narrator without reducing singularity either to "individuality" or to a determinate position within given social structures. In so doing, I have tried to emphasize the concrete particularities of each interaction, locating identity in processes of identification or the empirical articulations of memory, subjectivity, and discourse and performing the im/possible excess of any one self.[29]

The book inscribes in its form the emergent quality of performance, the possibility for birth story performances to draw reader/listeners into suspense—into a place where the meaning of birth, maternity, the female body, and raced, classed, gendered sexualities are at least temporarily open, up for grabs, subject now, primarily, to the rules of invention and protocols of exchange. Under these conditions anything can happen—including the realignment of primary social relations (Bauman 1977). The book charts a "carnal and vital topography" (Deleuze 1986:126). It writes otherwise atomized (anatomized) stories and selves into a shifting matrix, providing the subjunctive ground for "new political aggregates—provisional, uncomfortable, even conflictual, coalitions of bodies which both respect the concept of 'situated knowledges' and refuse to keep every body in its place" (Russo 1994:179). I have consequently transcribed the interviews in a simple, long-line verse or "ethnopoetic" style that is meant to reflect the rhythms, intensities, pleasures, and perversities of bodies (each to the other) that have their own—supplemental, complementary, contradictory—stories to tell.

Birth stories are viscerally relational. They constitute affective networks of social relations. They may thus contribute to the prospects for what Kenneth Plummer calls "intimate citizenship" (Plummer 1995). They may, more simply yet, recover erotics from the margins to the center of everyday life.[30] They may overwhelm discipline with pleasure and desire, rewrite birth discourses out of and into love, and charge mundane scripts with the real (corporeal) promise of making ourselves up over and over again, together, in performance.

CHAPTER ONE

Origins in Absence

BIRTH IS THE SIGN AND START OF BEING IN THE WORLD. It is the gateway of *presence*. Re-presented, it takes on a life of its own, grounding individual and collective identities, tying future to ancestral worlds, training *being* to the course of *what's been*, and guarding individuals, families, and whole ways of life against incursion by *difference*—by variation on a repeated theme, by challenges to the rule of *what's been* sedimented in the law of *what's done*.[1]

But what happens when a story begins in absence? When it takes its momentum from a gap, a break, a border space, or element of difference that violates laws of repetition and re-presentation even in the act of repeating, retelling, representing birth? What happens when "the boundary becomes the place from which *something begins its presencing*"? In this chapter I want to think about stories that are "ex-centric," that are not centered in presential histories, that begin their presencing out there, on the margins of what's been and done (Bhabha 1994:4–5).

The stories that follow relay absence. They originate in something missing—in Margaret's story: the conclusive test results that might have preempted a second trimester abortion, in Lila's story: the heterosexuality and asexuality required of what's generally considered a "normal" birth. The stories that emerge in each case rise up against the norms that deny their integrity, that prefer silence, conformity, and invisibility. In the corporealities of performance they break through normative reiteration into the time-space of terrifying and exhilarating possibility. They bend to the breaking point the comic-heroic norm of birth storytelling, making story answer to performance, performance to difference, and difference to its origins in absence, in silence, in the blank expanse of not knowing and *unknowing* and what remains impenetrably unknown. In so doing, they sound a tragic-heroic chord in birth story discourses and yet shift the tragic impulse from death or difference onto normativity itself. They slip such apparently fixed categories as death, difference, and normality into a performative framework within which death may be relived, difference transformed, and norms made the utterly provisional, undecidable byproduct of an endless process of becoming.[2]

****

Margaret called me on a reference from a mutual friend. In whispered, halting tones—checking repeatedly to make sure that no one overheard our arrangements—she asked to meet at my house rather than at her own or at some more public place. In her choice of setting and in the distance she maintained once there, Margaret seemed literally to be guarding her stories from intrusion, to be securing their borders and her control over their reception. She seemed to insist that the stories she would tell me were hers and hers *alone,* as if she were now making of the extraordinary loneliness she felt a virtue, a source of strength and resolute independence. Margaret sat on the living room chair, at a long arm's reach from the muffins and tea on the coffee table, at once trembling with anxiety and anger and practically daring me to cross the two or three feet between us. I remember especially how she left: she slid past me, out the door, leaving me without recourse to a "proper" good-bye or the satisfactions of intimacy that had characterized other interviews, including parting thanks, shy hugs, and brief gestures at meeting again. Margaret walked down the front path and away, her chin cocked—in embarrassment? indignation? pride?—taking her story with her. I watched her back. I wanted her to turn around. I like to think I saw her fingers wave at her side. But finally I had to acknowledge that her stories were of a body neither her doctors nor her husband nor I would ever fully know or be able to keep—a body I couldn't hold to my own codes or habits of conduct: a body that would forever elude control, if only in its capacity to name the means by which it had been controlled and then walk away.

Margaret began by briefly recounting her first births: an emergency cesarean section and then a surprising VBAC, or "vaginal birth after cesarean" (while the doctor was preparing for a C-section, insisting against Margaret's own advice that she wasn't "progressing," she pushed twice, only to send her baby flying into the doctor's unprepared bare hands). She then inched forward in her seat, leaning toward me—her face so bright now she seemed to have caught a spotlight—and began nervously, then fervently, to tell a third story: the story of a second trimester abortion, a potential birth cursed, it seemed, by normativity.[3]

Margaret and her husband had undergone months of prenatal testing only to gain enough information to make them worry about the health of the developing fetus. Repeated CVS (chorionic villi sampling) tests were "inconclusive."[4] A second amniocentesis indicated some kind of genetic abnormality.[5] But blood tests went nowhere, ultrasound imaging revealed a whole, working body, and, as Margaret says, "I just really felt deep in my heart that everything was fine."

Continued and repeated testing seemed to promise Margaret and her husband knowledge—not just empirical facts or so-called hard data but the story implicit in the data, the social drama in which those data are plotted: severely abnormal genes, abort the fetus; healthy, "good" genes, bring it to term. Testing promised *truths*—those little zygotes of science and culture in which an appropriate course of action could be mapped like DNA spirals in a family gene pool. As painful and as dangerous as it was, testing seemed to reinforce the notion that truth was out there—or, rather, *in* there—and only needed to be found.[6] In being revealed, moreover, it would reveal a kind of destiny. It would make one course of action or another seem as fated as blue eyes or brown hair. It would harden preference into necessity. Through testing, it seemed, science would certify moral choice.

In the absence of such a guarantee Margaret was left with a kind and degree of ambiguity that was terrifying, even terrorizing, in its complexities. She punctuated her account of testing, of the repeated "invasions" of her belly by long probing needles, by jamming the flexed fingers of both hands into her thick abdomen (covered now by a woolly sweater and the lycra stretch of black stirrup pants), as if into and through the uterine wall. Furious with the instruments and procedures that had repeatedly, painfully penetrated her body to no avail, she also seemed now to want to claw open her belly herself, to break through the uterine wall, to see once and for all this baby and its fate, to *know* what to do. Performing the whole story in a gesture, she railed against the opaqueness of her body. At once frustrated with its stubborn refusal to yield up the truth and confident that she'd heard its unproved and unprovable message, "All is well," she enacted in her own body the contest that would proceed over, around, and on it: a contest in which various half-blind, frail, and human ways of knowing would compete for its future.

But this was a contest no one would win. Motivated by absence—the tantalizing absence of conclusive proof of abnormality—it seemed that absence itself, in one form or another, would prevail: either Margaret would lose this pregnancy and child or, as in the story repeatedly impressed upon her by family and friends, her marriage would collapse, her other children would suffer for lack of attention, and the daughter she carried and longed for would meet with untold isolation and sorrow. She began by asking, "Well—how complicated a story do you want to hear?" and laughing, proceeded:

> Umm, well let's see—
> when Jonathan [her second son] waaaas . . .
> four months old
> I got pregnant again.
> My husband *did* not want the child
> *absolutely*
> *did not want* another child, absolutely, period, no.
> And I *did*.
> And so I just said, "Fine, fine this will be it. This will be
>   the last one.
> This will be it. This will be the last one. This will be the
>   last one. I promise there won't be anymore."
> And *he* was just saying, "You know it will probably be
>   another boy and
> you'll have to go to *all* these sports events, you'll hate it"
>   (*both laugh*).
> *Excuse me*: the weeeeaaakest excuses!
> the weakest excuses you could think of
> to convince me that I did not want this child.
> He *absolutely* did not want three children. And so—
> I went to
> get a
> CVS.

With Robert [her first son], I had
amnio.
With Jonathan, I had CVS,
and I drove from [a nearby city, where she and her family
    were living at the time] to [another urban area, three
    hours away] to have it 'cause I had a cousin who told
    me—
she's a physician's assistant—
she said, "Don't have it done in [the town where she
    and her family now live]. *Go*—"
because the rate of miscarriage resulting from the
    procedure is directly attributable to the skill of the
    person who is doing this.

DELLA: Really?

MARGARET: Yeah, and the one, the guy in [the city three hours
    away] has about a—ohhh, I've forgotten now—
but maybe he's
a one-in-a-something and the ones here are two-in-
    something
or two-in-a-thousand
or one-in-a-thousand, or one-in-a-hundred or whatever.
So we drove . . .

DELLA: That's a big difference.

MARGARET: Yeah, we drove [to a place three hours away]
for Jonathan. And then, when I got pregnant with the,
    uh . . .
after Jonathan
I just decided that I had two small children: there is
    no way I can make it [that far] for a day—
driving all the way there
then going through the procedure
then driving all the way back:
I'll just do it here.
Aaaand so I went in and had one CVS
and it was inconclusive.
Aaaand I went in and had a *second* CVS
and it was inconclusive. (They didn't get enough chori-
    onic villi or whatever . . .)
And so

umm . . .

this was like: big needle punches both times

well, no

let's see—

yeah: the first two times they did the chorionic villi
    sampling just like

through your uterus.

Then

they did an intra-abdominal one

where they punched a needle in there

and they *still* didn't get anything.

So this goes on for like—three?—three weeks

(*clipped*): You know they can only do it once a week
    because the risk of spontaneous abortion is
    so high.

So I called my cousin and she said (*sarcastic*), "I *told* you
    you should have gone to the other city!" And I said,
    "Well, you know, they're going to do an early amnio
    next week; thaaaaat will be fine."

So they did an early amnio.

Still no results.

This is like every week for—you know—a couple of
    months.

DELLA: My God.

MARGARET: And umm . . .

DELLA: Those are painful too.

MARGARET: Oh yeah, oh yeah. Aaaand
    especially because *each* time that they're *trying* to get
    the fluid
    they don't just do it just once—
    they try it four or five times
    while you're there.

DELLA: Oh God.

MARGARET: And (*laughs*) so umm, let's see, so:
    then they did the early amniocentesis—
    still inconclusive.
    So *finally* (*slowing*):
    when I was *about*, I guess, four-and-a-half
    to five months pregnant?

they did the regular amnio
which is about the time I guess that it normally
happens.

DELLA: Four-and-a-half?

MARGARET: Yeah, and
so then we got this phone call: "Well there's *something*
funny."
(*rapid, hard sarcasm*): "What do you mean there's
something funny?" "Well we want to do some blood
tests on you and your husband." So Stan is like,
"Oh it's my turn now to get poked." (*laughs*)
So . . . basically uhh
(*clipped*): there was some sort of a genetic abnormality,

but the horrible thing is that they *don't know what.* . . .
It could be something really minor, it could be
something really major and so that just kinda . . .

Oh wait, OK, let's go back:
when I said "OK, this is the last baby," and he's like
"Well, you know, we really shouldn't have a child, we
really shouldn't
have this baby. . . . Poor Jonathan's not even a year old—"
'cause I would have had two babies within one year—
and he's saying,
"You know, this baby is not even one year old, he's just
going to be lost, and he'll never get any attention"—
and all this stuff.
So umm, I say, "*OK*, you put your money where your
mouth is and go get a vasectomy. I'm sick of this! I've
got the birth control pills, IUDs"—you know, just
everything you could think of—and I said, "I'm just
tired of doing this. You were there too that night this
happened (*both laugh*)—so don't make me make this
horrible moral decision of . . ."
you know . . .
so, so
the deal was he would get a vasectomy
and I would

be able to keep this baby.

Even though he thought this was a *terrible* idea,
he was getting kind of used to the idea.
But then we went through all this horrible genetic stuff
    and then

basically there's no—
you know, they're doing this big gene mapping thing—
but basically there is no way to know what it is,
what the problem is.
And so there's just enough information to really, really
    screw you,
screw your mind up

(*changing the subject*): and umm, SO
at that point I had
a horrible choice to make because
(*sudden rush*): suppose that the,
that the child . . .
(*asserting composure*): *First* of all,
because of the sonogram:[7]
the heart was fine;
the brain was fine—you could see the little brain
    pumping!;
the limbs were *all there*;
so it probably . . . what does that leave?
something real *strange*
or maybe retardation
or it could be something really simple—
there's just no way to know—and so
the not knowing . . .
If they said, "Well, your child has Downs Syndrome,"
    then you say, "Well, OK, this is a given set of things.
    Could I handle that? Can I raise a child that has
    these special needs, yes or no?"
But the *not knowing*, you know . . .
and I had about a weekend to make up my mind.

DELLA: Oh God.

MARGARET: Because

ummm

after twenty-some weeks

it becomes illegal

to have an abortion

and the Ob/Gyn said they won't even do it *that late*, I'd
    have to go to [the local teaching hospital]

and then the people at the genetics thing said, "we have
    some news for you:

if you don't have it *now*, you're going to have to go to
    the maternity ward and deliver

this child" (*clears throat*)

and I have a friend who did that

so I knew I did not want to do that

I *absolutely* knew I did not want to do that.

Oh

this is also at Christmas and

right at holiday time

and my sister descends upon me without telling me she's
    coming (*laughs lightly*)

and my mother had a *heart* attack and

I had a lump on my breast—and

it was, like, *real* stressful!

DELLA: Oh my God.

MARGARET: So

I just really felt deep in my heart that everything was *fine*.

I *really* did.

But my husband just said, "*Look,*

what if this is a profoundly . . . you know, deformed or
    retarded child?

The child's *body* looks healthy; what if this child lives to
    be eighty? What are you doing to your other kids?"

So we disagreed, and we disagreed, and we disagreed,
    and we disagreed aaaand

I talked to some other

doctors

and to some other

friends

and my sister counsels a lot of special . . . kids—

handicapped kids and stuff.
And she said, "It usually ruins the marriage, you know."
She said, "It just—it creates such *havoc.*"
And she said, "*Don't,* don't have that baby."
You know: "Don't."

But at this point I was already *attached*
and bonding and it was like . . .

DELLA: Five months now.

MARGARET: Yeah
it was over half way there!
(*laughing and shaking with the effort to hold back tears*):

and I was crying, you know, I'll just have two instead
of three; it'll be alright; it'll be fine; it'll be fine and
so you know and . . .
I hadn't told anybody because we were waiting for the
results of the genetic stuff
and, plus: it was kind of a surprise anyway (*laughs*).
And I just thought I would let Jonathan enjoy being the
baby
for a while.

DELLA: Yeah.

MARGARET: Yeah. So,
finally, I just said,
"OK, OK [to an abortive procedure]."
'Cause I thought:
what if they make me go deliver this baby? [assuming
that she had made the same decision after the legal
deadline had passed and the doctors proceeded,
instead, with an induction of early labor]
I'll be around all these happy mothers with . . .

DELLA: You would . . . They would induce at five months . . .

MARGARET: Yes, yes. At a certain point—whatever the number of
weeks it [abortion] is illegal [here]—
it was creeping up real fast.
So
what they would do, what happens very often—because
people want to *know*, they want to do

an autopsy,
they want to know what is *wrong*
with the baby:
they just deliver
the baby
in the maternity
thing
and then they do an autopsy and and tell them what . . .

That's why they were telling me, "You need to make up
    your mind *now*"
because, as I said
I had a friend who had a
miscarriage
at about five and a half months
and she said
she just cried, and cried and cried and cried
because she was—
here she was,
she could hear all the babies going to their mothers
and she had to *see* the baby.
I mean, you know, she *delivered* it.
She saw the baby
she held it
and all this stuff
and I just said I can't do that.
I said, "Stan, I can *not* do that.
There's no way.
No way, José."
And since he'd had a vasectomy, it wasn't a question of
"We need to know what's wrong for next time."
You know, so . . .
but, I was bummmmed . . .
(*hard sigh*), because
it was a little *girl*
and I wanted a little girl *so* bad.

DELLA: Ohhhh.
MARGARET: So, yeah, that
    that was another thing:

coming so quickly after Jonathan,
all this other invasion, you know, and it not working,
and not working
and not working,
and me feeling like
everything's fine, everything's *fine*,
and, you know, them saying (*sarcastic*), "No it's *not*."
And I just . . . do I believe them or not?
You know. And so . . .

DELLA: Did they do an autopsy?

MARGARET: No
because they *don't*
if you have an abortion.
I guess because it's not
one piece of,
you know, baby. So umm. But it was so horrible.

I had to go and have
umm what umm
a suppository stick.[8] They put it in your uterus
to make you
dilate

and they do *that*
more than twenty-four hours ahead of time.
So the *whole* time that's in there, I'm sitting in my *bed*
at *home*
and I could feel this baby kicking, and I'm like,
"Stan I'm going to the bathroom and I'm gonna pull
    this thing out. I can't stand it, I can't stand it."
And I just,
I cried and cried and cried all that whole period and,
you know, after . . .
I mean: it's just (*drawing her fists up, fighting the tears*):
    horrible
and I think . . . (*hard sigh*)
I wonder, about it; you know, it was so *nice*
the first two times to know

everything's OK.
But I wonder
if it's really so good sometimes to know if . . . [presum-
    ably: if the test results are negative or inconclusive]
(*fast and hard*): What I would advise someone to do
    about that [prenatal genetic testing and/or abortion],
    I have no idea.

DELLA: But, uhh, it's so . . . tempting. I mean,
I would want to protect my kid too.

MARGARET: Oh yeah, but . . .
if it was good or bad . . .
I'll never know.

This was, it seemed to me, the story Margaret had come to tell. It seemed to be the last and yet the first story, the "original" from which the others now took their meaning. From its vantage I began to understand why the anger with which she related her second birth (the surprising VBAC) still seemed so raw, so untamed by triumph. It was anger for this lost child, anger fueled by desire, anger so hot that it burned open earlier wounds, that might—as Margaret insisted it had—wane but would never go away. I began to understand now that this absent child shaded every-thing Margaret said, that in its absence it was perhaps even more present than Margaret's other children. It haunted their births with possibility, with a sense of what might have been, had they been subject to the same scruti-ny with the same inscrutable results. She forgives herself the prenatal test-ing on Robert and Jonathan as she might a slight indulgence—"It was so *nice* / the first two times to know / everything's OK"—but goes on to worry about the implications of such knowledge when everything's not OK, sug-gesting that, to the extent that she finds genetic testing not always "good" or even morally neutral she is also bereft of the kind of authority that comes with believing, unequivocally, innocently, in the value of acquiring scientif-ic data and its implications for action. "I wonder / if it's really so good sometimes to know if . . . " she says, leaving a blank as wide as her own uncertainty about her baby's health, "What I would advise someone to do about that, I have no idea." Left, then, with less knowledge even than she had before she began this third round of testing, and less confidence in her own performativity, Margaret later indicated just how tangled abortion and birth were for her now. As she explained, weary with anger and loss:

> It [abortion] is sort of on a continuum with . . .
> birth
> and all that other stuff—
> because had I not . . . [imagined this outcome]
> because I was
> thirty-five when
> Robert was born
> and it [genetic testing] was available to me at each
>   [birth]
> but you know, I wonder, "What if I didn't know? Would
>   it have worked out OK or . . . not?"

What she cannot say, but what seems to boil up in the stammering pauses and vague allusions of what she does say (she actually uses the word *abortion* only once and then only to explain a procedural matter) is that her other births are now edged in guilt. They are framed not only by the absence of a third sibling but by their mother's broken desire ("I wanted a little girl *so* bad"), by her decision in the face of desire and hope and felt certainty to give up this life, by her nondecision, by what might as easily be called a failure as an excess of performativity: she acted, performed her self, within cycles of repetition that exceeded her control and effectively overtook whatever agency might otherwise have remained to her decision-making process. Exhausted by the endless (re)iteration of competing maternal norms to which she felt compelled, Margaret fell into a void of moral complexity and remained suspended there, caught in a net of betrayal, feeling as if, in wanting this child, she was betraying her family and marriage, and in aborting this child, "betraying this child for the other ones." She became, in the process, a ghost of herself, a figment of subjectivity, performing now the gap, the hole, the not-knowing and no-where to which prior performances assigned her.

Margaret is reluctant to blame anyone for the trauma of her own ambivalence. Having just passed her youngest child's first birthday and anticipating what would have been the due date of "the baby," she is circumspect:

> I think I'll probably always resent
> my husband
> because he didn't want the . . . he didn't want this child
> *anyway*—

and so it's like he got *his* way and I *didn't* (*laughing*).
You know, it's like those weird power things that
    people do.
Of course, he would never have wanted me to go
    through *that*
and he had finally decided yes, it was all going to be
    OK.
You know, so it's, it's not really . . .
it's just that irrationally you want to blame *some*one
or have some reason for this terrible thing to have
    happened
(*without rancor*): and, you know, I can't really blame the
    doctors, they're just doing what they're doing,
    you know:
what people want them to do.

Refusing to place blame, Margaret admirably refuses to become bitter. But she also lingers in the vestibule of her own guilt. She is, after all, the one who "irrationally" wants to "have some reason for this terrible thing." She is one of the "people" who, by her own assessment, makes medical practice go, whose demands lend medical staffers impunity—"They're just doing what they're doing"—and whose husband performed according to game plan—"It's like those weird power things that people do." In the end responsibility for the alleged "decision" to abort falls to her.

I don't want to suggest that Margaret should have or could have done anything differently. To the contrary, it seems to me that she is overburdened with agency in this scenario. Whereas other mothers with whom I talked scrambled to recover some agency in the birth process, fighting off if only by story a technological *coup de corps*, advancements in reproductive technology abandoned Margaret to her own "choices." With studied cool the doctors and counselors dispensed information-only: info-bytes, nondirective facts, facts without meaning or presumptions for action. Or so it seemed. As willing as Margaret was to read the abstract data assessments presented to her as further evidence of how little anyone really knew, she finally couldn't help but hear in its rising undertones a loud, resolute recommendation to terminate the pregnancy. In the absence of incontestably negative test results, from beneath the rumble of data and medical instruments, and against her own body's advice, emerged a statistically driven, moral mandate: "No," she reluctantly heard, "don't do it":

DELLA: Did you feel like they were
          leaning
          in any direction—
          I mean, were they encouraging at all . . . ?

MARGARET (*brusque*):
          No—and I think they . . . I think they *really* try hard
              not to.
          I think they really try hard not to, because they don't
              want to influence you because they know how big a
              deal it is.

          And there's the woman who was the genetics counselor
              who, like, *tells* you and holds up the little chart
              (*sarcastically*), "Now if you're over forty the chances of
              a Downs Syndrome child da da da . . ."
          And she
          was at the genetic testing place
          and she . . . she
          made a point of going *with* me when I had to go to the
              hospital
          to talk to the counselor
          about what the chances were and stuff.
          And I think basically what it came down to was
              numbers, which—
          what do *numbers* mean?
          There is maybe a 3 or 4 percent chance? of there being
              something severely wrong
          and then, when you get to be forty, it jumps up to about
              7 percent—
          and mine was varying more towards 10, 15, and maybe
              more, maybe *more*. So—
          but that's just, you know (*tossing it off*): that's just some-
              body playing with raw numbers; that doesn't *mean*
          anything (*laughs*)!
          You know what I mean.
          It's like: it starts looking real *bad*, but ummm . . .

DELLA: But it's still just so abstract.

MARGARET: But it doesn't *say* anything, yeah.
          It doesn't, yeah: it doesn't *do* anything.

Yeah. Sort of the way I felt about
the two
that I have,
I thought, "They're not going to have Down's
Syndrome." I just *knew* that they weren't.
And they *didn't*.
It was *fine*.
But that just frustrates me even more because I was so
sure everything was *fine*
and then it turns out not to be
probably. . . .

So . . . here's another case of me wanting to say, "But I
think it's OK," and they're saying, "No, with all of
our technology and stuff, we know it's not."

Silence also seemed to speak more loudly than words when Margaret's husband asked a doctor, "What really does this *mean*?" and he answered (as Margaret reported her husband's report) " 'Just don't, don't take a . . .' " The doctor's partial response was like the partial information Margaret and her husband received from the genetics counselors; it was enough information, enough advice, to damn the listener into completing the story in its own terms—to try to guess the riddle and then cling to its answer as if it were more special, more precious, if only because it was at first absent and mysterious: just don't, don't take a . . . *chance*. Hanging onto this unspoken "chance" are all the "horrible things" the doctor has seen under similar circumstances—the unspeakable deformities and afflictions that have followed from ignoring probability charts. In calculating this chance he enjoined Margaret and her husband to minimize risk, to listen to the various "what ifs" that clung to Margaret like pestilence and weigh them in a cost/benefits analysis disposed toward one choice: abortion. As if scientism and economies of risk must take up where science and testing instruments leave off. As if ambiguity were itself the enemy and must be cut up and cut out first by abstract, rational, and then by surgical means.[9]

This story seems to me tragic and heroic if only in the sense that Margaret's choice was not free—it was radically constrained by and to normative expectations; but, for all the pain and anxiety that followed in its wake, it might as well have been. Unlike Agamemnon at the fount, readying his daughter Iphigenia for sacrifice to the gods, seeking absolution for his ships as they unmoor for Troy, Margaret does not yield feeling to fate.[10] She does not become the stony pedestal on which the lamb is slaughtered. She is rather torn and torn again by "not knowing." She continues to live in the gap between desire and rationality, filled only with a horrible sense of their respective insufficiencies. She lives between ways of knowing, knowing nothing but that there is no knowledge sure and strong enough to carry her home. This story doesn't end. Its hero doesn't die or return triumphantly to an ancestral hearth. Telling this story to a stranger, Margaret continues to wander in exile from a home that, it seems, was never really hers:

DELLA: So . . . is there some way this whole thing could have happened
differently,
that would've been better?

MARGARET: I could have decided to take a leap of faith and just have the child.
I wanted to do that
and my husband didn't
and that . . .
I don't know . . .
(*choking back sudden, wrenching sobs*): I went to the dental school the other day and ummm . . .
I saw this *mom* and her daughter and she [the daughter] was like a teenager and they had their arms around each other and it was just like (*laughing*) . . . :
Aaahhhhhh!
But then, about five minutes later, I saw this very crippled little girl who looked like she was in a lot of pain
and I was like, WELLLLL (*both laugh*), you know: it could have been either way,
there's just no way to know.

The shadow figure, the image of the "very crippled little girl" that had trailed far behind Margaret's sense that "everything was *fine*," finally caught up with her, providing her with a strange measure of comfort: maybe she did the right thing, it could have been either way (it could have been *this way*). Each test deferred knowing along a course that required another test, that promised completion even as it deferred knowing and completion again, to another test or procedure. But when no neat sterile end could be found, myths of monstrosity filled in. Some combination of fear, revulsion, and pity at the prospect that her little girl might have been this "very crippled little girl" gave Margaret at least a moment's chance to stop wondering. To complete the deferral. In the end the futuristic technodrama renewed itself in the ancient (patriarchal) story of the mother who reproduces herself in a monster, whose own monstrosity (especially in the form of sexual excess) is realized in a child's twisted spine or shrunken limbs.[11] Performing within and against this narrative, Margaret saved both herself and her child from such unbearable and, maybe worse yet, unacceptable outcomes.

＊＊＊＊

In the classical epic, women and the territory they inhabit are the dank, monstrous, and mysterious obstacles the hero must overcome in order to be a hero. In being overcome, the feminine landscape defines the hero's triumph. She is the "plot-space" through which he must pass "to accomplish meaning" (de Lauretis 1984:109). The Medusa and the Sphinx—or, for that matter, their topographical equivalents: the Cyclops's dark cave and the dangerous narrow passage between Scylla and Charybdis—are the reason for and object of the hero's agency, the space that must be cleared before meaning and order can take the shore.

Several of the stories I heard were what I would call feminine rather than fully "feminized" epics. They did not correct male-driven heroics as much as they rejoiced in having survived them. In these stories women spoke out from the conventionally feminine role in which they were sometimes quite literally cast.[12]

Alternatively, several of the men I interviewed described feeling frustrated in their desire to fulfill the masculine role to which the "husband-coached" model of childbirth conventionally assigns them. For various reasons they felt displaced, dismissed, diminished next to the strapping image of the father/mentor invoked by the coach metaphor. In James and Kathy's case, for instance, James felt cut from the script, pushed out of the frame by the twin presences of Kathy and her sister, Beth.

I spoke with James and Kathy in a cramped hotel room that became stuffier as we talked (I was on a one-night junket in the city where they lived). They spoke in rough concert, Kathy from the edge of the unmade bed, James from the one chair in the room.[13] Each waited anxiously, graciously for the other to break, to pause, to attend to the baby sleeping fitfully in a car seat at their feet or to appease their three-year-old son Max (who valiantly occupied himself with a few small toys), before filling in missing details or supplementing the other's perspective with his or her own. They worked hard to keep the story of their second son's birth together, to twist its diverse parts into a single strand. But, the more they talked, the more futile the effort and the more brittle the story seemed. Eventually, their single story broke uneasily into two.

They agreed on this: whether by luck or design, Kathy's sister, Beth, arrived in town just in time for the birth of Kathy and James's second son, Aaron. Her arrival gave Kathy the impetus to tell James she'd prefer Beth's attendance during the birth. In the end James also attended the birth but remained on the sidelines, as it were, watching Kathy's joy in her sister's care, sensing Kathy's nearly ecstatic relief in Beth's deep massage, bearing her subsequent recriminations for not immediately "bonding" with the newborn baby, and feeling his own loss expand proportionately to her pleasure.

Their stories differ dramatically, however, perhaps most significantly in when and where each ends. Kathy's story resolves not with the baby's birth (as convention might suggest) but some hours later, with her and Beth up all night talking, remembering in tone and gesture years of playing together, sharing secrets after lights out, lost one to the other in the pleasure of their exchange, as much like new lovers as devoted sisters:

KATHY: The *end* of the story is:
after the baby was born
I was really completely elated, I couldn't sleep.
Beth and I just spent . . .
stayed up all night talking.
James was exhausted and went home. He . . .
again, this was like the *tradition*: when Max was born,
    James had to give a big lecture in front of hundreds of
    people the next day.
And the same thing when Aaron was born:
he had to prepare a big lecture and give it *that* day
having not had
really any sleep.
So James went home . . .

DELLA: So what time was it then that Aaron was born?
This was early morning.

KATHY: Two o'clock.
Two in the morning.
And then . . . James probably left not long after the
    baby was born, (*asking James*): right?

> Probably about three or so
> James was home. He went home.
> And Beth spent the night with *me*
> which was really nice.
> I mean, at this point they were *very* nice:
> they wheeled in a cot for Beth and, you know, we stayed
>   up *all* night *talking* and, you know . . .
> it was really great.

James' story ends differently. In fact, it barely ends, trailing off instead toward an indecipherable future. As he tells it, the birth was "a very dramatic performance of marital difficulties." It was a concentrated reflection in action of his marriage that, in turn, intensified its "difficulties." It (re)figured James outside his son's birth, outside his wife's affections, and, at first, distant from the child he'd much awaited. Telling it, reperforming it, he seems to walk just to the edge of grief and wait there, brightening with the last vestiges of hope, seeing and yet refusing to see over the edge of this particular cliff to his subsequent divorce from Kathy and his current fight to retain joint custody of his two boys. For James Kathy's devotion to Beth was if not the quake that destroyed the foundation of their marriage then at least an aftershock that secured its collapse. It left a hole simply too wide to mend. As James tells the story, he seems already to be free-falling, to be mourning an inevitable future moment when he crashes and crashes again into the disintegration of his marriage. Counterpointing Kathy's comic pulse, he writes a tragedy about to occur, about to be born, a tragedy without any kind of hero, whether masculine, feminine, or feminized. For James Aaron's birth brought with it a burgeoning absence. His story of Aaron's birth, moreover, opens onto an uncertain field of identity and action. As James observed midway through our interview:

> I felt
> ah
>
> well, I mean I felt involved in looking right at the baby
>   coming out
> you know.
> But, ah,
> but it was a little complicated—because Kathy and I
>   had had, uh disagreements

about *how*, about how this would *go*
and ah, so ah . . .
I was happy that *Beth* was there.
Because Beth was the person that Kathy did *want*,
    though Kathy didn't *ask* Beth "Would you come in
    order to *do* this"—it just happened that it worked out
    like that.

But ah,
but I guess my imagination of it was that it was
    something that the *two* of us should have done . . .
and the sort of *scene* that Kathy is describing,
this coaching kind of thing you know, I felt
ah, you know,
less than central (*laughing*).
But it was OK. I mean I didn't, you know . . . it's not
    that it
caused any problems really.
It went very well
and I was really glad that Beth was there and was able
    to help. And she really was a *big* help.
Ah, but I mean: you read all these books and so forth
    about it, and you know, it's this *couples* thing
and we knew before
going into it
that it probably wasn't going to be that for us

and, ah . . . so.

James's is the performance of a failed narrative. Reaching for closure
but managing to grasp only a vague ellipsis ("and, ah . . . so"), it suggests
not so much his failure to realize the hero's role in the conventional couples or husband-coached birthing script as the failure of the heroic narrative to sustain him in his designated role. Suddenly and, given the previous course of their marriage, apparently inevitably, the script changed.
This was no longer a (presumably heterosexual) "*couples* thing." James,
staunch in his alienation from the coaching "scene," was out, a moot point.
He was, as Kathy repeatedly noted, at home for what proved to be the climax, dropped from the script, not feeling at home at all but fulfilling a

"tradition" of exile, wandering in an-other's place, a stranger now to otherwise familiar norms of relation.

Another interviewee, Lila, also told what seemed to me a heroic story, a story of a radical choice that contradicted the "male model" of both medical and narrative practice. It also was a story that originated in absence, this time an absence produced not by loss but denial: the denial of lesbian rights to maternity and legitimate sexual expression. And yet Lila's performance of her story inverted the norm by making the absent present: by triumphantly claiming birth-rights against considerable opposition, formal and informal, by privileging sexuality in the birthing process, and by, in effect, feminizing the hero.

Lila and her partner, Megan, play out the alternative script. They both usurp the hero's role altogether (they set the course and followed it steadfastly) and transform that role into a distinctly feminine one, into a shared vehicle for an open, expansive, multidimensional exercise of love and desire. For Lila telling the story (as she ritually does on Rosie's birthday) is itself then a rite of extraordinary pleasure. It is a way of confirming and renewing their remarkable choice:

LILA: We reward ourselves when we get a chance to tell it again
          because of our perseverance, and um, um,
          plotting the way that we did it (*smiling*)
          and um, enjoying how much Rosie was wanted
          and how much she's still wanted and loved
          and feeling that that has *grown* . . .
          it's like *following* a course
          and not deviating
          and feeling real good about that.[14]

In taking the hero's part, Lila and Megan simultaneously fulfill and undermine it. They fill it and exceed it. They bust it open from the inside. The heroic role demands and exalts choice. To that extent, it suits their needs. But the controversial nature of the choice they make, the communal rather than individual stance enacted in it (Lila consistently defers to an inclusive "we"), the force of the love that flows from it ("enjoying how much Rosie was wanted / and how much she's still wanted and loved / and feeling that that has *grown*")—these hang below the cuffs, making the role seem an ill-fitting costume, outgrown and overworn, a little uncomfortable, even a little bit silly in its insufficiencies. In performing a role conventionally reserved for men, Lila and Megan both appropriate and parody its power. They perform its failure as performance to remain either gender- or value-fixed.[15]

For Lila Rosie's birth was a carefully deliberate act, a story written in the face of other stories that seemed to repeat, over and over again, like a scolding parent: lesbianism is an aberrant form of sexual practice and lesbian mothering is an intolerable transgression of heterosexual rights. These border stories and trespassing signs (masculine versions of the Sphinx and Medusa, marking out difference, securing one order by tracking its "other") surround Lila's story with fear and punishment—fear that lesbians will produce lesbians or gays, fear that lesbians will abuse their children, punishment for threatening masculine control.[16]

In fact, as Lila tells her story she seems to hem in grief and pain, briefly alluding to other stories, other plights, only to stitch them under the edges of this one. She twice excused the mess of papers and books covering the dining room table by referring to a workshop for incest survivors she was preparing for the weekend. Each time she did, her face darkened, her eyes turned away then returned brightly to the topic of Rosie's birth. She tucked her "failure" to conceive on their first try into another story, just as quickly opened and shut as her history of incest: "At the same time," she said, "a real close friend of all of ours died of AIDS and so I think it just wasn't the best time . . ." Recounting her daughter's birth, she deferred what she called "the hard part" (the cord wrapped around the baby's neck, fourth-degree vaginal tears, a difficult recovery) to a quick, final summary. Much of her story, moreover, was literally written in advance. It was rooted in two preemptive documents: a semilegal prenatal agreement meant to forestall the custody battles that would otherwise undoubtedly ensue should she and her lover ever break up and a carefully negotiated birth plan, intended both to protect and to honor the sexuality of all three of Rosie's new parents: Lila, her lover Megan, and their gay sperm donor, Eric. What Lila and Megan didn't anticipate, or couldn't anticipate enough to write it out of the script, was the extent to which their bodies would be punished through Rosie's: how a diaper rash would lead a caregiver to report them to social services for sexual abuse or how an early school teacher would laughingly reprove Rosie's claim to have "two mommies and two daddies!"

Lila and Megan relied on artificial insemination but bypassed clinical procedures through an ad in the paper ("Wanted: warm, fast swimming sperm") and the domestic, populist alternatives to medical instruments: an artichoke jar and a syringe. Told in Lila's soft undulent tones, this seemed an especially gentle raid on the dominant system, a mild *perruque* enjoyed as much for its simplicity as for its success.[17] As I listened to Lila, I could- n't help but think that, in their tactical maneuvering over and through a ground conventionally reserved for heterosexuals and medical experts, Lila and Megan were something like reproductive hackers. As John Fiske would argue, they "excorporated" the codes and equipment they needed to get into the system and, once in, showed the provisional owners of the means of (re)production just how weak its defenses were (Fiske 1993:197–198).

In this "localizing" effort they not only defied conventional, regulatory procedures and expanded the realm of their own control but shifted the operative social paradigm (see Fiske 1993:181–185). Suddenly the awkward corporate sterility of the sperm bank transaction took on a neighborly aspect: "Eric or [his partner] Dan—one would bring the sperm over / and Megan would help me inseminate it." As Lila talked, insemination began to sound a little like cooking dinner with friends. The structures implicit in medical institutions (centered in the doctor/patient dyad) and in hetero-sex, specifically the missionary work of heterosexual intercourse (reproducing itself in the nuclear family and patriarchy more broadly), fell away to a horizontal network of friends and references. With the support of this large and diverse community, Lila was more or less free to conceive on her own terms. She could perform both her sexual and maternal roles with equanimity, without fear of being upstaged by either men or machines (suggesting such a transcendence of heterosexual norms that her ninety- year-old Southern Baptist grandmother rationalized the birth as a kind of "immaculate conception").

In the hospital birthing room the center of power shifted according- ly—with dramatic consequence. After twenty-two hours of labor at home, exhausted and frustrated, "stuck" at six or seven centimeters, Lila finally went to the hospital. Having tried to ease her difficult transition period by relaxation exercises and meditation, her doctor (with whom they had formed a supportive pact) finally suggested an alternative to the artificial administration of the labor-inducing hormone, oxytocin (commonly known as pitocin or "the pit"): manual stimulation of the mother's nip- ples, a form of sexual stimulation intended to release the body's natural hormonal supply:

LILA: . . . so um, on the way to the hospital I had
back-to-back contractions
and that was just really exhausting, painful.

(*laughing*) When I walked in, my doctor said, "Boy, you
   look exhausted!"—
she looked like she was worried (*laughing*)!

So . . . she was *amazing*.
She did meditations with me . . . ?
and I slept in between, during my transition period: I
   slept between my contractions.
She was *really fabu*lous.
She was just
right there.

She knew our situation and
she had been *real* supportive all along
and she knew when I started trying
and she knew how quickly it happened and she, you
   know . . . (*imitating the doctor's strong voice*): "Hey,
   good work!" She had just been real good about it.

And um, so um . . . at some point
we had written up a birth *plan*
and we had asked that, instead of using the pitocin drip
   that we be allowed to use manual stimulation
at that point
if that needed to happen.
And that is what happened.
We needed to do something.
She had decided that—
her judgment was that I was really tired . . . ?
and to wait for
me to dilate more would have been
too exhausting and she said that, you know, we needed
   to either take the pitocin drip or do manual stimulation
and the midwife was there
and she really encouraged her.
The midwife was *very* experienced and
had done five hundred births and
knew a lot—and
(she was also a P.A. [physician's assistant])
and so *she*

encouraged her to

let us try that

and so um (*her voice breaking slightly*), *Megan*

did the manual . . . she did, um, manual stimulation of
    my nipples and it worked.

And so we didn't have to use

the chemical.

And it's like: that makes your body produce the same
    chemical that's needed to push you forward.

DELLA: Fantastic.

LILA: Yeah, yeah. It was real special.

DELLA: How did that feel at that moment?

LILA: Well, I was real inside myself

um, and so, you know, it was just like: I remember
    saying, "Meg do it right!" (*laughing*)

"This is gonna work!" (*both laughing hard*)

(*catching her breath*): And um, when our doctor said, you
    know,

"Lila, you get to choose who *does* this," and so,

you know, I told Meg to do it,

I think they . . . well, the people there that were aware of
    other things going on [Eric and another friend
    attending the birth] said that the nurses there were
    just like: (*imitating their look—eyes wide, mouth open,
    hands clapped to cheeks*) all agape! (*rolling laughter*)

DELLA: I believe it! (*laughter*)

LILA: And um, my choice . . .

At one point Meg was using her hands

and our midwife said

"Um, Meg, I think it would work better if you used your
    mouth,"

and so she did

and she was right.

It was just like, that was . . .

I think the amount of *suction*

or something

that needed to happen

worked better.

And she had known from her own experience—the
    midwife—that that's what needed to happen.

This part of the story was spare, even modest, in its detail. I felt as if the body of the story was half–turned away from me, so that I could *hear* but couldn't fully *see* the midwife prompting the doctor to suggest stimulation, the doctor encouraging Lila to choose a partner, Lila telling Megan to do it, the midwife suggesting Megan use her mouth, the nurses gasping in shock. I could trace the agency from midwife to doctor to Lila to Megan to the baby girl whose head soon tore through the stretched vaginal opening and whose body the doctor then hurried to wrench free of the umbilical cord wrapped around its tiny neck. I could feel an erotic power heating up across a circuitry of touch passed woman to woman, lover to lover, hand to body, mouth to breast. I felt as if I were for a moment inside a widening circle, the delicate threads suspending mother and child in a watery interregnum stretching outward, this time drawing *in* the lover, midwife, doctor, even the nurses standing aghast in the doorway (their mouths open wide), then me, listening in five years later, and now you.

This particular charge to the uterine muscles was sexual and sensual but never sensational. In neither its event nor narrative form was it structured by either a desire to see or a "desire to be seen" (Phelan 1993:18). Refusing the scopic plane of desire and conventional femininity altogether, this wasn't a show—but it was a profoundly transgressive performance. Through the synaptic relay of agency, through the embodied practice of sexuality, and through the visible but counterscopic enactment of lesbian sexual identifications, it violated exclusionary taboos, made a mess of the gridwork normally separating sexuality, maternity, and medicine, and transformed a masculine space into a radically heterogeneous one.

In reperforming it, however, Lila was very careful. Her use of the words "manual stimulation" alone seemed to sterilize the process of threat and danger. Clinical, latinate, abstract—the phrase made the process seem a procedure as cool and calculable as any other obstetric method or instrument. And yet, given that what's called "manual" stimulation here is both manual and oral and is more commonly either autoerotic (called "self-stimulation of the nipples" by what is currently the most widely read pregnancy handbook) or mechanical (a friend reported four-hour-long sessions, each divided into ten-minute intervals, on a hospital breast pump), the phrase also seemed oddly inaccurate.[19] It rubbed against the content of the story like rough fabric against tender skin. If anything, it signaled what *wasn't* being said, what remained hidden from view, what Lila didn't make explicit or "spectacular" in language. Combined with other, trace elements of medical discourse—references to segmented body parts ("stimulation of my nipples," "using her hands," "'if you used your mouth'"), an uneasy diagnosis of effects ("I think the amount of *suction* /or something / that needed to happen / worked better")— Lila's use of *manual stimulation* seemed to hold off the salacious or maligning viewer. It guarded touch and the whole-body consciousness Lila conveyed when she talked about stimulation making "your body produce the same chemical that's needed to push you / forward" and feeling "real inside myself" from exposure and attack. By performing her story at least partially within the discursive limits of the medicalized birth, Lila seemed to use medical discourse against itself. She appropriated its legitimacy to her own needs and lingered in the safety of its folds.

Carefully controlling what her listener *sees*, and indicating as much in the closed tones and tensions she conveys, Lila acknowledges the extent to which she and Megan transgressed norms of visibility in the process of birthing Rosie. In the birth, in fact, Lila and Megan made vigorously *present* what is usually as bracketed out of the birthing experience as death itself: not the mother's sexuality exactly but her sexual agency, her right and capacity to exercise sexual prerogatives, to perform her sexual identity, and to enjoy the power—physical and political—generated by such a hybrid/izing performance. To the extent that sexuality is acceptable in the birthing room, it tends to be either tamed to the business of procreation, buried under the cozy romance of holding hands (or, as is increasingly common in birthing hospitals, the promise of a candlelight dinner), or controlled by derision and surveillance. As various critics of hospital birthing have shown, an accumulation of minor adjustments—the mother's supine position, the hospital gown draped im/modestly over her upper body, the sheet hiding her lower body from all but the doctor's eyes, her lower body disconnected from feeling and thought by an epidural, her gaze diverted to the schoolhouse clock on the opposite wall—channel her sexuality toward one end only (literally, the bottom line): the efficient production of a baby.[20] The mother's body is, in effect, reconstructed within the time-space zone of Cartesian rationality. Like the magician's assistant, she is cut in two, her head, brain, mouth, and voice divided from the mechanical labor of her lower body. She is encouraged to go along with the trick—to experience her body as a contest between rational will and stubborn flesh—by the promise that in so doing she will be able to "control" her own birth; she will be able to overcome her body's lascivious pain and irreverence by force of thought. She will be able to make this birth as clean as the magician-physician's cut—rational, controlled, unembarrassed by such sexual corporeal excesses as exposed and leaking breasts, nausea and vomiting, bursting amniotic fluids (often turned yellow-brown by the baby's own shocked shit), excrement pushed out with the baby, blood that made my hospital room look (as one night nurse so tactfully put it) "like a slaughterhouse."

In this scenario sex is aligned with what the anthropologist Mary Douglas calls "matter out of place," or what we commonly call "dirt" or "dirty" (Douglas 1966:35).[21] It is the marked violation of the hospital space, a performative transgression: an active assault on the hospital's immune system by a foreign body (see Ward 1992). Shameful, animal, and inappropriate, it is also in this space unhealthy—and so subject to cure largely by containment. To the extent that it is invoked in the birthing room—by the hospital gown that inevitably slips and reveals what its presence nonetheless says should be covered or by a physician's friendly "dirty" jokes—it is also dismissed and displaced, reduced to an object of attraction and repulsion. In this way it takes on a pornographic aspect—enhanced, as several mothers suggested to me, not by "gazing" at the mother in any particular way but by ignoring her altogether and watching TV. Next to presidential debates, the World Series, news of the gulf war, or even the Flintstones, the birthing mother is at best a secondary spectacle—and one now subject to the kind of locker-room joking stereotypical of men-watching-men compete. As one mother reported it, her doctor took a break from whatever game he was watching with the father-to-be to perform his own pumped-up sexuality on her birthing body. She laughed as she retold the joke with which he framed her birth experience: "Why do Southern women have so many babies?" the doctor asked. "Because it takes them so long to say (thick Southern drawl) 'Noooooooooo!'"

In other words, the hospital birthing room doesn't need "manual stimulation" to make it sexual. It is already fraught with the implications of birth for a woman's sexuality. A pregnant body is a sexual body. Whether accurately or not, its expanding belly declares "this woman has had sex"—above all making the conspicuous alignment of sexuality with maternity vexing for a Western, Judeo-Christian culture divided by identification with Eve and adoration of Mary.[22] Western maternity typically entails silencing the sex in which it (like the child born) originates. By, among other things, keeping the pregnant (and nursing) body at home and making it wear clothes that either hide its swelling curves or dress them up in the innocence of girlish pinks and bows, we conventionally cut maternity off from its flush and fertile "other": sex.

But sex isn't as much the problem here as the havoc it wreaks on a clear sense of division between the sacred and the profane. Maternity must be purged of sexuality, it seems, because we cannot tolerate their confusion. To the contrary, through "manual stimulation," Lila and Megan not only entered a space in which the sacred is profane and the profane sacred, but they resignified sex. They performed beyond the compulsive order of sexuality, re/iterating sex as excess and agency. Here, in word and act, in Lila's particular restoration of the radical sexual agency entailed in "manual stimulation" was the sex that "made" this baby—that sent it, finally, ripping down the vaginal canal and into the hands of the waiting world. Here too was the defiance of difference—whether the presumed and regulated differences between maternity and sexuality or between lesbian and hetero-sexuality—that *made* the difference, that broke through difference into abundance. Here was a superoriginal moment—a moment that did not so much violate as exceed norms of (re)productivity, a moment filled to overflowing with love, care, pleasure, and potential. When Megan put her mouth—the most confusing and multivalent of bodily orifices (located on the public side of reason, the mouth is both animal and intellectual; it produces and consumes; it tastes and chews what it takes in; it expels speech, spit, and vomit)—on Lila's breasts (the most explicit markers of femininity, now ripe with maternity, lolling in the liminal midzone between head and belly), she released into the birthing room a kind and degree of energy that simply couldn't be contained—or even named—by "normal" means. Here, the neither/nor ambiguity that Margaret suffers (neither desire nor rationality would yield up a decisive truth) becomes a both/and plenitude of many truths: both mind and body, both medicine and sexuality, both utility and pleasure conspire here to make a baby, a lesbian mother, a family out of friends, and a heterogeneous world-space in which normativity falls away, at least for a few carefully guarded moments, against the rising force of love and desire.[23]

The lesson of Lila's story, for me, is not that lesbian sex is better than other kinds of sex but that by recovering performative sexual agency to maternity, maternity gains strength and power—the power even to overcome masculine heterosexual preferences for this-or-that (categorical differences and singular truths). In telling her story, Lila testifies to the unique capacity of bearing, birthing, and mothering to initiate not only a new life but many new lives, to give life to multiplicity and community in the name of "enjoying how much Rosie was wanted / and how much she's still wanted and loved."[24]

Lila's story also suggests what the feminist theorist Julia Kristeva calls the "homosexual facet of motherhood" generally, the extent to which in and through birth the birthing woman is drawn into a deep libidinal relation with her own mother, a symbiotic relation in which she is both mother and child and her mother and child are as much a part of her "self" as she is of theirs. For Kristeva:

> By giving birth, the woman enters into contact with her mother; she becomes, she is her own mother; they are the same continuity differentiating itself. She thus actualizes the homosexual facet of motherhood, through which a woman is simultaneously closer to her instinctual memory, more open to her own psychosis, and consequently, more negatory of the social, symbolic bond. (KRISTEVA 1980:239)

Kristeva imagines the maternal body as a preconscious, preverbal (pre-Oedipal) space—a space before language or "social, symbolic" control, in which the "self" rediscovers its continuity with "others." Maternity is not thus (as psychoanalytics more aligned with conventional forms of femininity would have it) a matter of regression or return.[25] Rather than a lapse in identity, it is the realization of identification with others on the corporeal ground of "feeling, displacement, rhythm, sound, flashes" (Kristeva 1980:239–240). It does not entail "going back" to an edenic origin but achieving at the margins and in the cracks of social structures pure originality—or what Kristeva calls *jouissance*: the excessive, transgressive power that follows on the (dangerous) *pleasures* of maternity.[26] Maternity is not, for Kristeva, an individual event or condition. In its satisfaction of semiotic desires and its promise of *original* pleasure, it is rather a pervasive and continuous threat to the grammars of everyday social life, a rumbling series of shocks to the norms and rules of difference by which we call all kinds of female pleasure (whether specifically sexual or symbiotic) bad. As I understand Kristeva, the maternal body is a rupture in the social fabric always already about to happen.

In Kathy and James's case, the maternal body expanded, in effect, to include Beth and to exclude James. In Beth's arms and through her cradling, kneading, encouraging work, through the twin labor of her own and Beth's bodies, Kathy found a new beginning, a family of origin/ation, a family remade in the tender yielding of one girl-child to another, one mother to another, two sisters to each other. Against this deep, familial, homosocial bond, the heterosexual contract on which Kathy and James's marriage was based (strained as it already was) could barely hold up. James in fact spoke as if he were reading the world through its holes and around its fraying edges.

In Lila's case the break was more volcanic, rising as it did against the flat surface of medical and sexual convention, igniting what might be called a "homosexual matrix" in which Lila, Meg, and now Rosie's home, the local medical center and health service agencies, and the hundreds of friends, acquaintances, and admirers attending an outdoor concert at which Rosie's birth was announced (barely moments after it happened) were now entwined.[27]

Still, I hesitate at the threshold of Kristeva's theory. As much as I am drawn to its revolutionary promise, I withdraw from what seems Kristeva's willingness to abandon particular women to a general "maternal body," to privilege feminine "psychosis," and so to cede ego, choice, and deliberation to cultures of masculinity (surely, Margaret's anguish and Lila's pleasure in their respective, carefully deliberated choices would proscribe such concessions).[28] And yet I remain moved by Kristeva's sense that maternity is a utopic force, drawing together women, mothers, and their children—male and female—in the deep and sensual renewal of their lives together. Among other things, Kristeva's sense of the maternal body as a site of joyous identification suggests a framework for understanding the refrain that seems to join all the stories I heard into a single chorus—a refrain that usually went something like "Now I understand what my mother went through" and echoed from one story to the next in expressions of an often urgent desire for female birth attendants.

This desire seemed sometimes desperate (Margaret's longing for a friend or advocate who might relieve her of the sense that she was alone in her struggle), sometimes romantic (my own expectation that a female doctor—by virtue of being female and a mother at that!—would be "naturally" more sympathetic), sometimes intensely familial (a labor-and-delivery nurse I interviewed put off pushing for an hour and a half until her mother arrived from half-a-state away), often charged with the heart-pounding, pulsating sense of pleasure and play, ecstasy and energy that Kristeva calls *jouissance* and that a few of the women with whom I spoke dared to call erotic.

The erotic charge that, for these women, lit up the performance of giving birth also seemed to light up the stories they told about it.[29] Many of the stories I heard were not specifically sexual but, in the telling, were filled to overflowing with the kind of intimacy, excitement, pleasure, and passion that articulated itself in and through the birthing body they hailed—a body that, in being given, *gave*, that exceeded its limits in joy and strength, that managed, like Demeter retrieving Persephone from hell, "to go and get the baby on another planet / and bring the baby back."[30]

And yet, listening to Lila again, and to James and Kathy and Margaret, I recall many birth stories that hedged on the erotics of birth or that conformed more neatly to conventional comic plots. I think again about how violently my friend inveighed against the power of birth stories to silence his story, to turn out his story into a lack, an absence. And I wonder how much the performance of birth stories reproves not only stillbirth and miscarriage (the oohing and cooing over a new arrival shaming death into hiding) but infertility (the oohing and cooing teasing desire into desperation) and homosexuality (the oohing and cooing boosting the "miracle" of hetero-sex). I wonder to what extent I have in fact complied with a heterosexual norm by telling birth stories. To what extent do I and other birth storytellers, in telling our stories and subjecting ourselves to others', contribute to the rising cult of the bio-baby—at the same time that new technologies make mom-and-pop baby making as obsolete as the corner grocery? Does taking pleasure in our respective lines of (re)production exclude alternative family formations—gay/lesbian families, adoptive families, families without children, single-parent families, families born in difference? Do we, in telling birth stories (squeezing in details at the store, in the parking lot, in between our daily affairs) implicitly rehearse one answer to our children's question, "Where do babies come from?" reiterating without sufficiently re-marking an answer whose own gaps and absences resist the more demanding forms of origin/ality, the claims of maternal performativity that Margaret and Lila's stories represent? Hearing the child's question, the plea for final origin, I find myself answering despite, or, perhaps, to spite myself: "A man and a woman *lie together* . . ."

CHAPTER TWO

Narrative Rites

"Push!" screamed Amy.
"Pull," whispered Sethe.

—Toni Morrison, *Beloved*

The "one" to whom I speak has moved in with me, deep within me . . .
—Nancy Mairs, *Voice Lessons*

MY DAUGHTER WAS BORN BLUE. Within hours of her birth, she was taken by rescue squad from the hospital in which she was born to a near-by teaching hospital equipped to respond to acute respiratory failure. I had just started to fall asleep, to fall into sleep, finally giving in to the resident's assurances that she would be "fine," when I awoke to a curt knock on the door. The same resident now informed me that she had "bad news" and that the rescue squad was on the way. My husband and I were instructed to wait. There was nothing we could do at the other hospital but wait—and we might as well do that here. The baby wouldn't be officially admitted for hours. We watched the paramedics rush the incubator bubble down the hall and then received a stream of doctors and phone calls, some with explanations, some with none, some with welcome silence. At around 6 A.M., we left, first for home, to see our two-year-old son, Nat, waiting there, and then to the hospital. What followed were days of washing hands, slipping into sterile gowns, gripping the side of the metal crib, reaching for Isabel through the net of wires and beeping machines that seemed to hold her, to cradle her, as I couldn't. Caught in that limbo of wires and tubes, she seemed strangely safe. We waited.

Like all the other parents and family members marooned outside the neonatal intensive care unit—the NICU, or "nikky," as we came to call it, each of us apparently oblivious to the others' routines, I walked to and from the nursery, to and from the cafeteria; sometimes I circled the elevator tower just for a change of pace. And when it was free I huddled in a gold-colored vinyl recliner in the far corner of the parents' waiting room, turning away from the pasty glare of the fluorescent lights, the smells of cleanser and take-out food, the rubber heels squeaking on the tile floors just outside the door, the everyday sounds (chairs banging, low laughter, paper bags being crushed into trash) that filled the waiting room and that seemed so awfully out of place, so patently, unrepentantly *ordinary*, toward the small spiral notebook that, following all of the good advice of all of the birthing handbooks I'd read, I'd dutifully brought with me.

I wrote in it, frantically now, buttressing the present with the immediate past, writing Isabel's birth into this place of uncertainty, inscribing its ragged, unkempt promise into and against time. It was as if by writing I could hold off time itself; I could hold on, at least, to the weak provisions of waiting. I refused to "jinx" the careful balance in which Isabel seemed to rest with expressions of either hope or dismay. In the face of all the misery that seemed to wait on all of us waiting there, confidence seemed dangerous, even shameful. I wouldn't take up the nurses' generous litany: "She'll be OK." And yet writing Isabel's birth, I seemed to contract myself to a secret agreement, to a secret I kept even from myself: she would be OK. Filling my notebook pages with the mess of Isabel's fast, crazy birth, I wrote in fits of anger, irony, exhilaration. I pressed the pen on page after page, scrawling over two, three lines at once. My neck ached from trying to write half-sitting up, half-lying down. I wrote what I knew:

> *everything out of sync*
> *lights on and off*
> *contractions on top of each other*
> *quirky Dr A keeps joking about the bill at the pizza parlor he'd been called away from.*
> *could never get ahold of the situation*
> *nurse never really there—and when she was, she wasn't. reprimanding.*
>
> *was she just dying to come out? strong and blue, covered in vernix—but relaxed. We know each other.*
>
> *never getting an adequate position. nobody offering to help—sensing or hearing my unwilling pleas for help*
> *Alan talking—digging relentlessly into my back*

countering the rockets of pain that were throwing me up and across the bed

like a giant fish hook in my back
Alan tells me he could see the spine pressed out by the baby's descent

and then a voice raised for children: "I am going to have to check your
cervix while you're in a contraction"
the nurse never came into direct view, was always leaving

everybody talking to me while I'm blind—increasingly frozen with
pain. Even Dr. A trying to extricate himself from my grasp: "you're
breaking my hand and if you don't let go I won't be able to deliver your
baby"
asking about tearing last time—snide: "you must have been delivered by a
nurse-midwife"

at 8 cm, the baby like a giant golden ball pressing at my lower rectum,
insisting that I help it out—"I have to push!" to the air, Dr. A, again,
from an odd corner of the bed, 1/2 turned, 1/2 dismissive, almost taunt-
ing : "I can try to fold back the cervix . . . " and then: "don't push or you'll
tear the cervix"—a vague sense of threat

disentangling from the mess of fetal monitor bands and cords I never
wanted to go to the bathroom to shit

then the order to move my legs "square up your knees" the giant operating
lights suddenly descending from the ceiling behind Dr. A's head. where am
I?? my head won't talk to my legs—can't make them move—I can't breath
for the pain

flopped around, childlike "it hurts" "oh boy" "ow"

blue rubbery wet doll on my chest—I wish this gown was off. much to my
amazement: you are blond!

then the dumb transfer to the postpartum floor. "go to the bathroom" (I
have nothing to void) and emerge to a waiting wheelchair. they pile my
stuff on and we get wheeled—eventually—to a dumpy old hospital room.
at least it has a window. drab small. no room for Alan much less bags. I

think: a sure prescription for postpartum depression. if you didn't have it before, this would do it—

These notes mean what they say. They describe Isabel's birth. They also mean what they explicitly don't say—that in that birth her life was at risk. They also mean by saying—by using or *doing* words, often against a representational grain. As seductively transparent as they may seem, these words are not windows onto the world of birth. Rather, by creating the impression of a reality before words that words reflect back to us, they create that reality itself: they project the terms by which birth is and should be understood; they intervene in cycles of representation, refusing to take for granted the status of the birth experience as such (as if this is the way things are and so must be); they resist what John Fiske calls the "tyranny of the indicative" or of *what is*, writing away from a referential real into *what might be*, or what I would call, from a performance-centered perspective, a *possible real*. In their rampage across even these carefully typeset pages, they are tied to those rituals of meaning and magic by which words are dangerous because they have effects, because they make worlds and beings previously unseen, untouched or even unimagined real, because they mediate being itself (Fiske 1993:119). In the spirit of the (much contested) difference between what the language theorist J. L. Austin has called constative and performative utterances, they do not refer to so much as they perform Isabel's birth: they insist on the fulfillment of her birth in life.[1]

Writing these notes was for me a kind of diversion. It was a way of ignoring and biding time. But it was also a very literal way of *diverting* time, of directing it toward one mortal outcome rather than another. Reading these notes now, I thrill to the strange vitality of their rough random form. I feel again my old stubborn insistence that things should have been different, that time itself should do things *my way*. I look down to see my hands balled now into fists; I feel my jaw clench and face stretch into a mad grimace; I am suddenly banging back, punching out these words on the keyboard: *make her live*, rehearsing again the claims I made then, and make over and over again, everyday, in different ways. If there was ever a beginning in the word, I want it now as I did then—when my own struggle with time through words was not as far as I was tempted to think from the prayers that the families gathered in the waiting room often offered together. I was once or twice invited to join in these prayers but hung back, performing, instead these, my own rites of protection.

Back home, memory and context conspired to produce a different story. I began to (re)write Isabel's birth for her this way:

woke not feeling well—not quite right: achy, head heavy. Alan knew: same as last time—attentive all day, encouraging me to lie down.

we have a babysitter for a last date. wouldn't have gotten out at all if I hadn't wanted to see a friend's direction of Haydn's Creation. *A balmy fall night. As we walk back towards campus from dinner, I feel the pull of the huge pancake boggy moon hanging just above the trees before us— full yesterday, it is yellowing and frayed at the edges, about to drop. I feel the same way—a deep heaviness pressing on my pelvic floor. I remember actually reaching down to hold you up as we walked—like a big sack of groceries—dismissive of the contractions I casually timed (about 15 minutes apart) during dinner—I'd seen the same pattern so many times before.*

at campus—lots of middle-aged people in trenchcoats and heels gravitate toward the sedate but brightly lit concert hall. Hill Hall, 7:30. As I head up the steps and just glimpse the sparkling foyer, I feel a warm, thick gush of fluid breaking from my body, filling my shoes. Laughing, I turn to Alan, just below me: my waters broke! a man beside me on the stairs, stops, staring, not knowing what to do—as I stand there giddy with pleasure. Alan goes into motion—scooping me along, talking constantly, mapping out the way to the car. I skoosh beside him, still laughing, the waters bursting in waves as we walk.

I insist we go home to get the bag we never got to the hospital last time. I try to calmly change from my favorite pregnancy dress—gold tapestry pattern, a swirl of fall colors now soaked—into a shirt and sweatpants as we make our respective phone calls. Alan arranges for a neighbor to stay with Nat. I talk to Dr. A (the doctor with whom we arranged the birth plan). He doesn't remember us from yesterday and says wait until the contractions are 7/8 mins apart; they'll call him from the hospital. Recalling another doctor's warning to get going at 10 mins apart (given that you were early, I was already dilated to 3 cm., Nat was fast and this was my second, suspense was high . . .) and bowing to Alan's anxiety about getting to the hospital, we packed up, kissed Nat goodbye, and left.

The contractions go from about 8 mins to 2–3 minutes apart in the car. They begin to hit like bullets in my back. I am still gushing water. We get lost! We miss the exit, take the next one, and can't find our way back on. Alan's narrating signs to me; I want to laugh while I try to breathe through contractions. I have no idea where we are. In a clear moment, I see a blur of bright green signs in what seems another language . . .

We get to the hospital. Alan drops me at admissions and goes to park the car. I balance against the desk while the admitting nurse calls up to Labor & Delivery; with perfect deadpan sarcasm, she holds the phone away from her ear: "I have to ask: are you sure your waters broke?!" then answers for me, "She's sure!" Alan reappears; while they take more info, we wait for the wheelchair, I hug into his shoulder, this time laughing and crying, excited and relieved: it's here! we're going to have a baby! everything is going so fast.

The nurse races through the halls. The grand arrival. We emerge onto the floor, into a huge bright blue room. beautiful but cold.

At this point the story breaks off. What began with such narrative promise—the prosaic moon, the ironic attempt to hear the *Creation*, our classic performance of getting lost on the way to the hospital, the romantic crescendo, the dramatic, even operatic "grand arrival": all disintegrates into a mess of images and moments. For several weeks after the birth I didn't want to—and couldn't—tell what happened next, except in formulaic phone messages: *"waters broke on the steps of Hill Hall, on the way to the* Creation!" *"went from 5 to 10 centimeters in 1/2 hour!"* and the occasional, muffled, *"It was not a good experience."* I felt foolish for having let the event get so far away from me and embarrassed by what seemed the very storylessness of it all. So crazy, so unhinged. Narrative norms at once buoyed me up and failed me.

Nancy Mairs describes the autobiographical past as a "dream house," a locus of "mystery and desire," an imagined as much as a remembered place through which the writer and reader pass, pass each other, and find each other in the correspondence of their imaginations: "I invite you into the house of my past," Mairs offers at the start of one memoir, "and the threshold you cross leads you into your own" (Mairs 1995:11). I felt exiled from my own "dream house." It wasn't that I wouldn't or couldn't tell my story exactly, but that I felt I had no story to tell, no story worth telling, no invitations to offer.

And yet I had to press what few keys I had to the lock and push the door open because this dream house, this locus of "mystery and desire," was not fundamentally mine at all but Isabel's, or ours, a reciprocal composition, as Mairs suggests, of Isabel's history through mine. Isabel made this plain, insisting, as did her brother (do all children do this, I wondered?), that I literally perform her birth over and over again, each time as if for the first time. She would hide under a mess of blankets or in a laundry basket or in some other womblike structure and I would have to *push and push and push* until she popped out from wherever she was and I held her and I was, according to script, *so happy* (sometimes she and Nat wanted to play at the same time and I birthed in stereo, often for several repetitions at a shot; sometimes they surprised me by emerging as various baby creatures—usually, fortunately, small domestic animals).

The house of this past is marred and worn with each retelling, suffering its worst injuries with the onset of each birthday season. Each year, as we mark time by Isabel's age, reinstalling her origins in the pleasures of balloons and cake, the story gains more and different details, new and different intensities. At first I confirmed the rudimentary bits Isabel practiced early on:

> *Yes, Daddy and I both held you and we were so happy* (this was something of a fictional truth or a true fiction imported from the story Nat would tell of his own birth; it is true and not true: there was no time for this actually to happen, for happiness to intervene before anxiety took over; but we did both hold her briefly, at some point, before relinquishing her to doctors and machines, and our happiness rushed like an underground stream into the pool of love in which, telling the story now, I bathe her).

I checked her story against the various "textbook" versions she had already learned:

> *No,* I say, *you weren't all cleaned up before I held you* (having to side with her brother on this one)*; you were covered in the goo and blood that protected you while you were inside me—before the doctor took you away because you were BLUE.*

I embellished her retellings and my weak memory with imported dialogue and action:

> *That's just the way you always were,* I tell her, *after she has passed through one of her wild rages: even when you were in the hospital and the nurses tried to do something to you, like wash you or fix something, and you would*

arch your back and turn bright red from head to toe and scream so loudly I thought something was horribly wrong and the nurses would smile and hold you up like this (balancing an imaginary head and bottom on two outstretched palms): *"No, that's just the way she is!" and they smiled because that meant you were the healthiest, strongest baby there.*

And eventually fell into memorializing the continuity of the past with the present (flattering their ragged discontinuities) in the simplest, most mundane turns of phrase:

That's one of the songs Daddy and I would sing to you when you were in the hospital.

Or: *That's just like the moon on the night that you were born.*

As we perform these stories, small and large, encapsulated in a phrase or elaborated in action, back and forth, across the threshold of "mystery and desire," Isabel's self is centered in a past she knows only because we tell her. We perform her. We make and remake her foundational sense of identity and being in the world in the reiteration of stories of her origin, in stories whose originality is renewed in each (re)telling.

Birth stories can force winter roots. Their power to stake identity in origins of their own making is perhaps nowhere more fully expressed than in stories that are repeated relentlessly, without change, across time. Unflinching in the face of time, these stories lack the sense of contingency, possibility, and play typically associated with performance.[2] They are stories hardened by repetition into fact. They are performances distilled down to the texts of human lives.[3] As such, they cast a pall of immutability, or what often passes for fate, over parent and child alike. The origin story that is sedimented in history as fact tends to naturalize a given reality and, in turn, to fix its characters in set identity or "subject" positions. It may be used, as one woman said, "to point out to me that I should be doing one thing or another that I wasn't doing." Sometimes told sardonically (whether by the parent or child), as if laughter were the only way around beginning life in three days of excruciating labor or in *"how much we went through to have you . . ."* or in the indignities of birthing under welfare and hospital regimes or, worse yet, in the shadow of loss (one friend's mother repeatedly recalled her first child's stillbirth: *" 'The doctor had told me not to have another one . . . I was too small' "*), it also often evokes a deeper sadness, a sense of being overwhelmed by one's origins in story.

The child sees him or her self—what she has been and can become—in her birth story. The birth story may thus displace what is commonly considered the "birth itself" as the origin of understanding and self-becoming, generating through its own forms—however open or closed, however constrained to obligation or risk or pain they may be—a *reality-effect*: a child, a self, an identity produced and reproduced within given narrative terms. But insofar as narrative is the field of production, it is always vulnerable to variation and reinvention: it is the dynamic ground of a *possible real*.[4] It charges the self and its (internalized) others with the possibilities of becoming (otherwise). It does not reflect an originary moment as much as it mirrors back and forth images of the mother and child, mother and mother, self and other, in the act of looking, each into the other, for the grounds of their respective identities.

And yet what each can see is limited by what each can tell; what each can tell is limited by the claims of other narratives, other selves on the telling self. What each sees is always already a mirror image—not the self but an image of the self, refracted through an-other's story. The harder each looks, therefore, the more elusive an essential self becomes: "I" becomes the "you" that "I" tell.[5] Subject and object fold into each other and, in turn, into a cacophony of family, religious, and social histories: "I" disappears into "you," into the stories at once told by and about "you," into the mixed blessings of (re)creating the self. On the other hand, "I" / "you" may disappear altogether. The distinctive, expressive force of the telling self may fade into a sense that there is no story to tell, that there is no tellable story or that there is no story worth telling other than those that are always already told: those that are preauthorized by replication within the normalizing discourses of obstretric practice or those that are, for whatever reason, pressed flat into the pages of family memory.

The story self is a double self—a self doubled up in the pleasures of performance, in the sensuous entanglement of self-subject and self-object in the art of *making memory*, doubled over in memory of lost selves, divided against itself in the performativity of answering to others' stories.[6] Isabel's birth story is my/her story. It is, like other birth stories, a double image of the mother and child, cast now into an ongoing struggle to co-create selves. The child inhabits the mother's story, shaping it from the inside out. The mother's story is pregnant with the child's own, even as it recalls first rites of separation (pushing, expelling, cutting, weighing, testing, wrapping, removing). What Nancy Mairs has said of autobiographical writing echoes literally through birth stories: "I don't see how anyone engaged in self-representation can fail to recognize in the autobiographical self, constructed as it is in language, all the others whom the writing self shelters," she says; "The not-me dwells here in the me. We are one, and more-than-one. Our stories utter one another" (Mairs 1995:11). The "I" in the birth story, the mother-"I," is a shelter, an enunciative context, a rough hold for multiple others whose stories overlap as they unfold, each into another's, each exceeding the other's in the process of making a self-story that is at least twice told. The mother-I is not, or, is not only, a foundational subject: she is also transformed in the double act of speaking and being spoken; she is subject to the very performativity of her own speech acts, becoming herself, becoming *the one who tells*, in the act of telling what simultaneously becomes, however tenuously, *her story.*[7]

The *one who tells* is "always reworked in . . . enunciation."[8] The mother-I tells what/as she becomes. Subject to the contingencies of reiteration, she slips from the privileged place of identity or *being* into the rougher ways of identification or relational *becoming.*[9] In this light the birth story is always already a double story, redoubled in exchange between a parent and child, between siblings, between parents, between mothers, between a child and unspoken others, between a child and the self she might become. At least two selves are reworked in any single, variable repetition. At least two selves are poised each to become an-other, to become each other, even each other's other, in the invitation to enter the house of another's past and, in so doing, not only to cross into one's own but to cross one's own past with another's, in what is ultimately a performance of desire: an enactment of the kind of desire that drives the interplay of memory and imagination, history and invention, repetition and revision,[10] that transgresses boundaries of self and other, present and past, that draws bodies together in words echoing back and forth, "mouth to ear," ear to ear, belly to belly.[11]

My stories are concentrated in images that are keyed to larger narratives: Isabel felt *like a giant golden ball* (a *golden globe,* I sometimes say now). The contractions hit *like bullets in my back.* The nurse was condescending, *reprimanding. dumpy old hospital room. born blue. the* Creation! *got lost!* These were first words. But they are also old words. Imports. Clichés. Citations. Images and formulaic themes worn smooth with use. They are and are not "my" words in the sense of original or unique, but they are the tokens of origin I carry now as close as muscle to bone.[12] They constitute a cellular memory. They have slipped, like so many snapshots into the sleeves of family albums, into the place of memory, recalling *what might be* in the image of *what has been.* Holding me there, at the threshold of "mystery and desire," they seem to have a life of their own. They make "me" even as I tell you Isabel's birth, even as she ("not-me") becomes herself in my new/old words.

These words, hard and fixed as they may seem, tied as hard and fast as they are to expectations for class privilege, to the easy deployment of high culture references (*the* Creation!) and narrative competencies (*like a golden globe, born blue*), to heteronormative complacencies (*Daddy and I both held you and we were so happy*), to a patriarchal family history lined with embarrassment and shame (condescending, *reprimanding*), and to popular comedies of getting lost, getting through, and finally getting a baby, nonetheless also signify the *disturbance* of narrative at its root, in exchange. In even the most rudimentary acts of telling, these stories, these words are always already partial, contingent, loaded, cut through with other words, stories, and histories.[13]

In the mid-seventies Nancy Chodorow offered an incisive critique of the discursive reproduction of the woman as mother that she called the "reproduction of mothering." Wondering why "women mother daughters who, when they become women, mother," Chodorow concluded (1978:209):

> The sexual and familial division of labor in which women mother creates a sexual division of psychic organization and orientation. It produces socially gendered women and men who enter into asymmetrical heterosexual relationships; it produces men who react to, fear, and act superior to women, and who put most of their energies into the nonfamilial work world and do not parent. Finally it produces women who turn their energies towards nurturing and caring for children—in turn reproducing the sexual and family division of labor in which women mother.

Adrienne Rich echoed Chodorow, ascribing more insidious implications to the duplication of the mother in the daughter under the rule of the Father (1986a:243): "A mother's victimization does not merely humiliate her, it mutilates the daughter who watches her for clues as to what it means to be a woman. Like the traditional foot-bound Chinese woman, she passes on her own affliction. The mother's self-hatred and low expectations are the binding rags for the psyche of the daughter." Rich offered, to the contrary, images of Demeter rescuing Persephone and Persephone saving Demeter by being rescued. Each, Rich argued, realizes herself in the other, in reconciliation with her "lost self"—her mother/daughter, her other/same. Appealing to the classical myth of renewal and rebirth, Rich turned the primary identification of the mother and daughter in patriarchy inside out.

For both Chodorow and Rich, however, the woman as mother is bound to reproduce herself in her daughter. Both reinscribe the "reproduction of mothering," projecting a kind of copybook model of identity that does not account, for instance, for what Carolyn Steedman calls "not-mothering." By not-mothering, Steedman does not mean, as middle-class moralities might suggest, choosing not to have children or being a "bad" mother—by failing to "bond" with a newborn, for instance, or committing some form of neglect. Rather, for Steedman, not-mothering describes a reproductive line skewed by the working-class daughter's suspicion that her relationship with her mother is not primary, that it is tightly bound up with class, and that class structure troubles patriarchal domination in such a way as to divide, rather than bind, the mother and daughter in their respective positions of exile. For Steedman (1986:88–89) histories of working-class children suggest a fundamental displacement of gender by class:

> Accounts of mothering need to recognize not-mothering, and recognizing it, would have to deal in economic circumstances and the social understanding that arises out of such circumstances. I think that my own mother's half-conscious motive in producing me was the wish that my father would marry her, though I did not understand the economic terms of my existence until long after my childhood. However, it is clear that many working-class children have understood these terms, quite precisely, and have developed an understanding of themselves in that light. Nineteenth-century girl-children of the 1860s, for example, interviewed by parliamentary commissioners, demonstrated that they knew themselves as workers as well as children, knew precisely what they contributed to a household economy.

Not-mothering (re)produces (girl-)children not as mothers but as workers, as means for their mothers to get husband-providers, as financial burdens, as participants in a household economy. The child who cannot gain primary affirmation from the mother whose gaze, whose look, is directed elsewhere is reproduced as *refusal*: "the refusal to mother, the removal of the looking-glass [the child's mirrored-self], reproduces refusal." Unable to see herself in her mother-self, to renew her self-love in her mother's love for her, the little girl becomes divided against herself, a half-self, a figure of alienation and lack, unable to satisfy a mother who refuses (who is unable), for whatever reason, to be satisfied by her.[14]

Steedman offers an important corrective to the collision of biological and discursive reproduction in Chodorow and Rich. For Steedman the reproduction of *not-mothering* results in a history of painful refusals that nonetheless suggests a politics of dis-identification, of nonreduplicative generation.[15] The reproduction of refusal or not-mothering is inherently unstable. It disturbs middle-class patriarchies with histories of lack, dissonance, exclusion. In the end, refusal, the knife in the heart of the girl-child, becomes politically strategic: Steedman withdraws her story from history. She refuses the seductions of narrative altogether, beckoning the darkness to which her story, once told, however, can never fully return (144):

> I know that the compulsions of narrative are almost irresistible: having found a psychology where once there was only the assumption of pathology or false consciousness to be seen, the tendency is to celebrate this psychology, to seek entry for it to the wider world of literary and cultural reference; and the enterprise of working-class autobiography was designed to make this at least a feasible project. But to do this is to miss the irreducible nature of all our lost childhoods: what has been made has been made out on the borderlands. I must make the final gesture of defiance, and refuse to let this be absorbed by the central story; must ask for a structure of political thought that will take all of this, all these secret and impossible stories, recognize what has been made out on the margins; and then, recognizing it, refuse to celebrate it; a politics that will, watching this past say "So what?"; and consign it to the dark.

Refusing to celebrate the "secret and impossible" stories of her childhood, Steedman asserts its irretrievable loss. She at once rejects the romance of recovering it (like Persephone to Demeter, daughter to mother, mother to daughter) and reproduces the refusal to which she was born.

Lingering in Steedman's dusky "So what?" I want to suggest that telling birth stories (when telling, as performance, means that they are always already fading into darkness) disrupts continuous lines of duplication and descent. They are sites of horizontal interaction, layered in refusals, in "secret and impossible" histories, in defiance, resistance, silence, replay, relay. They triangulate me, you, Isabel (each of us haunted, inhabited by multiple "others") in what Nancy Mairs calls an erotics of memory and imagination: in the "bone house"—or the rough-house cross-cut—of body memories that holds identity somewhere between stories heard and stories told, between stories told and telling stories. The reproduction of maternal identity falters against the contradictions and contingencies of birth stories in performance. It loses the smug assurance it gains by identification with patriarchy, relieving women as mothers from responsibility for either holding their daughters to a primary identification with their reproductive capacities or liberating them by impossible mythic powers. This is not to say that birth stories are not, as I have indicated, fraught with discursive complicities. It is to say, rather, that in and as performance birth stories hold out the possibility of breaking continuous lines of (discursive) inheritance, of founding new origins of being, of making *possible* selves, and making possible selves *real*. Bypassing narrowly reproductive for productive performances of self/other, birth stories refuse what Steedman calls the performative "compulsions of narrative." They slip identity from apparently fixed social positions into living, shifting, difficult, and yet often exhilarating processes of identification, suggesting different, if not altogether new, modes—even structures—of knowing, being, doing, and becoming.

My grip loosens. I surrender my fists to finger play. I don't tell Isabel as much as she tells me—producing in my memory/imagination of her both the pleasures and devastations of being told, of telling, of not speaking at all.

Daughter/Mother: Beyond Reproduction

Rachel's mother died of cancer when Rachel was in her mid-thirties, some time after she had married and moved with her husband, John, to a home outside of Boston and just over a year before Rachel became pregnant with her first child. Soon after her mother's death Rachel found herself in a bitter court battle with her mother's same-sex partner, each seeking what they felt were due rights to what little there was of Rachel's mother's estate.[16]

The legal battle rehearsed old antagonisms. Rachel's father, an unemployed actor at the time, had left Rachel's mother when Rachel was three, performing his version of the old vaudeville gambit: he went out for a pack of cigarettes and never came back (until he showed up at Rachel's wedding some twenty years later, wielding a baseball bat for mock protection). Rachel's mother came out as a lesbian when Rachel was in her midteens. Rachel was living with her mother at the time but never got along with her mother's lover. They just didn't like each other; they were jealous of each other; Rachel was angry. Her mother finally felt pressed to take sides and, in the end, asked Rachel, at sixteen, to move out.

Over the intervening years Rachel came into a sympathetic understanding of her mother's life:

I mean, she just lived such an anxious life,
for so many reasons, you know, manic-depression, the
physiological side of it, and being gay and . . . just so
many things that she just, in her lifetime, in her time
had to deal
ah (*sighs*), with: single mother, raising a child. Working
    way
under her potential. All these things, which is where I
    get my lack of
. . . ambitions.

She was a brilliant woman! I mean, she was offered a
    prestigious college
scholarship, you know.
Chose to go to a big-ten university from a
    small town,
Jewish, anti-semitism, she grew up with.
You know, all that, everything, getting hit with,
And parents who were very hard on her.[17]

Of her death, Rachel offered: "I think she just finally said, 'I've had enough.'" But for all the sympathy Rachel could muster, for all her identification with her mother's own lack of self-love and emotional upheaval, in the end her mother once and for all refused her clamoring need for attention and love, her need to be the primary motive in her mother's life as a mother. As Rachel said:

That's what hurts, 'cause it's like, Mommy, how could
    you leave me?
You know, I'm your baby, you know.
That's what I just . . . I feel anger.
How could you do this to me (*whispers*)?

When the court battle erupted, Rachel became the "baby" again. And, again, she was in an old, hot competition for possession of the mother/lover. The daughter and lover each turned now to the eyes of the law for a surrogate *look*, a confirmation of their respective claims to the rights of heterosexuality and homosexuality, legal and common law marriage, kinship and partnership. The case drew Rachel into a defensive identification with her mother that, in turn, inflamed her sense of blood rights. She was the daughter, after all. She would be a mother. She would (re)produce her own mother in herself as a daughter becoming a mother, as she had been trying to do for six years, in the last of these through various fertility treatments. The daughter wanted her mother to want her and she wanted to be a mother, to have the opportunity to satisfy her own child's desires in the flash of returned, maternal *looks*. (Once Rachel knew she was having a girl, she tried out possible baby names by imagining herself at the foot of the stairs, calling out this name or that, as if it were dinner time or time for school; she would look up, one hand on the banister, to see her daughter run to the landing at the top of the stairs in order to catch her name and to return her mother's awaiting look. The name that seemed to secure this moment, in which the mother and daughter's looks were most happily locked, was the one she would eventually choose.) At once the baby and the mother, the daughter who would be a mother to her daughter, Rachel became entwined in a politics of reproductivity that finally led her to devote her final award in the legal suit (the full sum of which was divided between the lover and the daughter) to a college fund for her mother's as yet only imagined grandchild (Rachel saw herself intervening on her mother's behalf, doing perhaps not so much what she would have done as what she would have liked her to have done; as she later said, "It's going to her grandaughter / She's going to be able to give her granddaughter this")—and to begin the first of three rounds of in vitro fertilization.

Despite putative success rates of 15–20 percent, at the time a total of some 380 babies had been born by in vitro fertilization. Much to everyone's surprise, Rachel's third try worked. Two of the five eggs returned to her uterus had apparently worked their way into the uterine lining (one soon dislodged), leading Rachel and John to expect twins. Annie was a "miracle" baby—not only by all scientific accounts but within the mystique of maternal reproduction that favors look-alikes, that grounds the authority of blood relations in lines of resemblance.[18]

At birth, and even more so as she grew older, Annie looked and acted eerily like Rachel's mother. As Rachel tells it, it was Annie's strange likeness to her maternal grandmother that, among other things, confirmed the miracle of her birth:

> I can't believe (*whispering*) that she
> was almost never here, you know, that I just . . .
>
> Not that I would ever not have been a mommy,
>   because I

know that we would have adopted. We would have had
a child.
I was not . . . I knew that we would have children, you
know, but ah . . .
I just, I, I didn't know. John had more faith.
But I, I wasn't sure, so when I do look at her now I
think
(*softly*) I can't, I just can't believe she's here.

And I can't believe how much she looks like my
mother!!
And my mother just died, and here she is, and it's a
girl, and
it's my mother's smile!

Through all this Rachel had never fully reckoned with her mother's
death. It was only when Rachel had her baby, when Annie seemed to
answer Rachel's desire to be the daughter become mother, that Rachel first
and finally realized her mother was gone, gone forever, present only as an
imaginary figment of what she might have been. In the middle of what
turned into a four-part interview between me, Rachel, Rachel's husband,
John, and my husband, Alan (the conversational play shifting un/pre-
dictably along gender and marital lines), Rachel recalled the moment her
mother's absence hit home:

RACHEL: And everybody came to visit, and then finally the last
            visitor left, my aunt left, and I thought, wait a minute,
            there's one more person that should be here.
            Where is she?
ALAN: When was that? How soon?
RACHEL: I would say like within a couple weeks, you know.
ALAN: A couple weeks.
RACHEL: And then it really started to hit, and I would just
            cry in the shower. And I was just, you know
            I mean . . . just . . . : you're a wreck.
JOHN: Yeah, yeah.
RACHEL: Hormonally, just ah, the microwave's been on too long.
DELLA: (*laughter*)
RACHEL: Oh, it was wild.
            But then that finally subsided, and, you know,

you can sort of get back to normal.
Normal, whatever that is again.
But, yeah, I just, I remember I kept thinking,
well, if she, I remember thinking privately to
myself, well, if she doesn't show up . . . for this

She really did die.

She really isn't here. You know (*louder*) what I mean.
You know what I mean. I kept thinking maybe she's
going to call someday, maybe she is really somewhere
else. If she isn't here for this . . .
I know she's not here on this, on this earth anymore.
She really is gone.
And, that's the final proof.

That was it for me.

And it had to move on from that point, you know.
You know, Alan, it had to move on.
I did think that, yeah.
I kept . . . I gave her one more chance, leaving the chair
for Elijah . . . waiting.
You know, you leave that chair and . . . you think,
and no, no, no, she didn't, she really didn't come.
No card . . . no phone call. Not even a phone call!
(*laughter*) Nothing.

DELLA: What, how did you feel then?

RACHEL: She doesn't write (*laughter*). She doesn't . . .
              But she died (*laughter*).
JOHN (*deadpan irony*):
              Yeah, the dead don't write.
RACHEL (*indicating what her mother might have said*):
              "Do I have to draw a fucking picture for you?" (*laughter*)
ALAN: Having a hard time, the economy down, the dead,
              they can't, they can't afford to travel.
RACHEL (*laughing*):
              Right (*everyone laughs*).

ALAN (*deadpan*):
> The mail service.

RACHEL: Not good. (*uproarious laughter*)

Basically, her mom just didn't show. Didn't even call. Didn't lead much less follow the ritual call to gather around the new mother, to initiate her into the rights and obligations of maternity by coming to see the new baby, to witness her presence in the world.

Suddenly, the vertical line of reproduction—daughter to daughter to daughter, mother become mother become mother—for which Rachel had, in court, in medical clinics, in her marriage, fought so hard, broke. There was terrible grief in this break, the kind of grief reserved for the failure of life itself to answer the child/mother's call, whether from the bottom of the stairs or from the top, grief ringing with the many losses and refusals that had preceded this final reckoning. But this grief came in the form of bawdy, raucous, (ir)reverent laughter. The uncanny diversion of the mother's look from the daughter to her lesbian lover in life became, in death, a source of absurd pleasure. The divisions that had for so long been animated and maintained by legal wrangling finally just folded in on themselves, collapsed into what is ultimately Rachel's story of the undisciplined, the uncontrollable body—the body that dies too soon, the postpartum body run to riot by hormones, the lesbian body, caught between lover and daughter, suspended in charges of deviance and neglect, the mother/daughter body compulsively replaying the rights and rituals of heterosexuality, the carnal, passionate, disorderly body honored in Rachel's story by both solemn tribute and obscene carnival parody.

Remembering her mother's death, invoking her absence in the immediacies of performance: Rachel moves with extraordinary precision from an abstract recognition to the embodied realization that her mother's out of here. Here was the final proof her mother had died. Not a coroner's report or funeral oration. Not an obituary. Pure and complete absence felt in sharp contrast to others' presence. Beginning outside the story, prefacing the immediate scene with summary—"And everybody came to visit"—and then slipping inside, asking now, as she apparently did then, "Where is she?": in the course of our conversation, Rachel's recollection of her mother's death becomes at once the defining fact of her recent past—"She really did die"— and the generative principle of her, our shared present: "She really isn't here." And just as *then , there* becomes *here, now* in the act of telling, "I" becomes "you." Her own devastation becomes general, common: "I was just, you know

. . . you're a wreck." Identifying with me and others who've suffered what seems the same bad joke—the body's adolescent rebellion (out all night and drunk on hormones) at exactly the moment the new mother most needs it straight and stable—she gains a comic foothold on death. She fights back against the trickster body, laugh for laugh, good joke for bad, deflating the power of postpartum hormones to reduce her to a "wreck" by comparing them to the legendary vissicitudes of everybody's favorite home appliance: "Hormonally, ah, the microwave's been on too long."

But with a short pause and ebb Rachel returns to the same point from another angle, shifting now from the spectacular grotesque to the sublime.[19] Against all odds Rachel had given her mother one more chance. She'd kept the door open. She'd stayed death with hope. She recalled contemporary psychologies of "denial" to the folk tradition of leaving an empty chair for Elijah—the reluctant, Old Testament prophet—at the Passover table, just in case he should pass by and want to stop in and, stopping in, herald the messiah: "I kept, I gave her one more chance, leaving the chair / for Elijah . . . waiting / You know, you leave that chair and . . . you think . . ." What "you" think, for a moment, in this ancient performance of hope, is that maybe this seder will not end in ritual anticipation of "next year," that maybe Elijah will follow that breeze coming through the open door, that maybe the waiting cup of wine and place at the table will entice prophecy into reality, and turn expectation and desire into eternal blessing.

Ironically, Elijah is also the guardian of newborns, called by the rabbi or mohel at the Jewish circumcision ceremony to protect the infant placed in Elijah's "chair" (usually lined with a prayer shawl, a tallis) from evil spirits. At the seder, the bris, or on the synagogue bimah before the sacred arc holding the Torah, the chair is meant to invite Elijah to give up his reluctance and to perform the miracles and prophecies from which he, like Jonah, shied.

But "no, no, no, she didn't, she really didn't come": her mother never took up Elijah's place; "She really did die." As I listen again to this phase of our conversation, I can't help but feel that Rachel's not only telling us about having realized this before but is realizing it now, having held off the "final proof" until now, here, in the company of friends, holding it to her, cradling it to her, as if she were once more setting a place for her mother at the Passover table, this time with a new baby in her arms, finally shutting the door after a late night chill reminds us that neither her mother nor Elijah has come through its inviting frame. And just as the celebrants around the table will repeat the same ritual next year, miming their hopes and blessing their desires all over again, so too I think will Rachel's performance of this story always reopen the door to her mother's life—if only, as she does here, to let the rabble in.

What happens after this appeal to sacred tradition? Descent. Deflation. Crude celebration of death in the terms of the living—or is it life in terms of death? Turning Elijah's absence into a burlesque of social protocol (he was, after all, expected), "No card . . . no phone call. Not even a phone call!" Rachel falls hard, still laughing: "nothing." A single line explodes into a four-part, elliptical riff. Suddenly death becomes being stood up at a really good party (ours):

RACHEL: She doesn't write (*laughter*). She doesn't . . .
            But she died (*laughter*).
JOHN (*deadpan irony*):
            Yeah, the dead don't write.
RACHEL (*indicating what her mother might have said*):
            "Do I have to draw a fucking picture for you?" (*laughter*)
ALAN: Having a hard time, the economy down, the dead,
            they can't, they can't afford to travel.
RACHEL (*laughing*):
            Right (*everyone laughs*).
ALAN (*deadpan*):
            The mail service . . .
RACHEL: Not good (*uproarious laughter*).

The image here (the dead as bad correspondents) is so impossibly bad, so irreverant, as to amount to hammering extra nails into the lid of a coffin. Basically, the joke goes, it's so hard to think of the dead as suffering a recession or bad mail service that they must be dead and gone. On the other hand, if current technology is such that you can have babies without sex (if we are postsex), then surely the dead should be able to call up from heaven or the grave and at least tell us they're dead! In the end the joke is on us, the living, who are so indebted to frail bureaucracies, delicate technologies, and social protocols (at least call if you're not going to show up!) for life that we might as well be dead. In the name of life we are apparently regulating ourselves out of existence. Less joking about death than enjoying death's joke on us, this is pure carnival: intoxicating parody, base, banal, regenerative laughter, a sideshow revival of death and sex—the ultimate signs of corporeal life—in the onrush of cyborg birth, death become life by rites of grotesque pleasure.[20] The dead-end, run-on jokes, the raging laughter—together they evoke a past crashing head-on into the perverse perfection of the "no-where"/u-topic present Dick Hebdige describes:

> There's nowhere else but here for us. No other time but now. This is all there is and it's enough to be getting on with. It's not so bad. In fact it can make us laugh. The realisation can produce laughter—not the artful snigger, or the hollow, savage laughter licensed "beyond the fringe" or amongst the avant garde, but something closer to a belly laugh: a pregnant laugh that might help to usher in a new order. (HEBDIGE 1988:239)[21]

Belly-born, this is Rachel's initiation into motherhood—not the righteous passing of the baton from mother to daughter for which she might have wished but the sensual, aggressive embrace of her mother's life in death. By upturning the pieties and proprieties normally associated with both life and death, she dies into mothering, she initiates new life—her own, new-born role as a mother without a mother, the power of our rude and vital bodies (now aching with laughter) to exceed rules of decency, and even the nearly palpable presence of Rachel's mother who would joke about anything, even get up again to tell us she's gone, screaming out from the other side (through her daughter's body now): "'Do I have to draw a fucking picture for you?'" if she thought it would get a good laugh.

****

John and my husband, Alan, were old college buddies. When Alan first met Rachel she was in her early twenties, living and working in Cambridge. She ran with a theatrical crowd, Alan tells me. Fast-paced, witty, loud. He couldn't keep up. When I first met her in 1985, shortly after Alan and I were married and on the cusp of John and Rachel's tenth anniversary, I too felt overwhelmed—as much by her extraordinary energy as by her extraordinary beauty. Her high cheek bones and jet black hair seemed to burn with desire and possibility. She seemed on fire. I remember standing a bit out of her way, not knowing exactly which way the sparks would fly, as she swept from room to room, fixing things up, joking, hosting.

It was only after my first child's birth in Boston in 1989 that Rachel and I became more than old friends by marriage. I'd never felt such pure need as I did in the wake of Nat's birth—and Rachel met that need with a kind of tenderness and aplomb that I simply had never known before. I can still feel the waffle-weave of the thermal blanket and the thin nylon of the hospital stocking cap (each gently marked and softened by her own use nine months earlier) that she brought when I complained that Nat wouldn't sleep. I can still feel the mattress bend and the brass frame shake as she climbed into my bed one morning—both of us dank with sweat and leaking milk—so that we could nurse our babies together.

This interview took place one year later at my home in North Carolina. John, Rachel, and their daughter, Annie, had come down to celebrate Nat's first birthday. Anticipating this conversation, we'd talked throughout the weekend about our respective births—in fits and starts, in flurries of comparison—"Did you do that? No, we didn't do that, we did this," recollecting the same kind of talk we'd exchanged (always one eye elsewhere, one ear out for a child somewhere) in Boston a year earlier.

In some ways the interview is the fruit of all that talk; in some ways it is only the residue, the trace left behind; in other ways it is a discrete event, confirming Samuel Schrager's sense that an interview is not "natural" conversation, that it is artificial, and that, as such, it provides "a new context for the telling of mainly preexistent narrative" (Schrager 1983:78–79). John and Rachel had clearly "storied" much of this material before. They had rehearsed it to themselves or shaped it into ringing narratives for others— even to the point of informally naming episodes ("the thing with grandma") and referring others to folk and literary genres (one omen story was "like an Indian folklore story," another was the "last little bit of drama"). But this was no more a simple repetition of past performances than it was a simple repetition or report of the past. Especially heightened moments in the process of the "progressive structuring of detail" that makes up most retellings, these set pieces only piqued our pleasure in what was artificial and artful in our interaction, in what was not natural at all except insofar as this conversation marked and magnified the artifice in everyday speech—the craft, play, composition, improvisation, drama, true fictions, and fictional truths—as well as the potential for (re)combining all of the above and more in the *performance of possibilities*, in the narrative process of making what's possibly true or what's im/possibly bad or good palpable in the sensuous immediacies of performance, whether that performance occurs in the apparently "natural" run of everyday conversation or in this, its mirror version, the interview.[22]

For all our rehearsal that weekend and during the preceding year, the interview proved to be—as it did on so many subsequent occasions—a stage on which the participants performed their histories as if for the first time, as if they were *hearing* those histories for the first time and, in the process, rediscovering and remaking them, emerging into the stories out of which the interview arose. Not only did John and Rachel conjure worlds we'd never touched before but we held and circled those worlds with a kind of sensuous pleasure that made us glad the kids were upstairs, asleep.

We were downstairs—Rachel, John, Alan, me, braced between the demands of children and hunger, sprawled across the floor and couch. The microphone seemed to hold us accountable—to ourselves, to each other, and to the meaning of birth for each and all of us. It intensified and amplified what now seemed a sudden encounter, each to each. Pushed off the plane of pedestrian chat into something like midair acrobatics—in the glare of the spotlight, in the moment between falling and flying: what now, here, would we make of all this? Feeling a slight sheen of sweat breaking out before the urgent claims of the camera, feeling the heat of something like glamor, something like honor, what we feared would be inhibiting self-consciousness became reflexivity: the kind of expanded consciousness—or double awareness of who we were with and for each other at the very moment of telling about other times and places—that comes with playing audience to one's own performance of self, life, and history. Making up (for) birth in story, trying to do it better, to do it one better, to outdo pain, loss, chaos, contradiction, gaps, boredom, banality, and even the beauty that is so beautiful because it passes so quickly in narrative form, we performed ourselves performing—sometimes simply marking what and where we once were, sometimes becoming ourselves all over again and so becoming *different*.

* * * *

John and Rachel began by distinguishing the in vitro (or intrautero) procedure from GIFT (gammin intrafallopian transfer), explaining that the latter, because it involves returning the fertilized eggs to the fallopian tubes rather than directly to the uterus "simulates more of a natural pregnancy" and so tends to be more successful. Because Rachel's tubes were completely closed off, she and John couldn't use GIFT. But, to compensate for whatever gap there was in the simulacra of in vitro, they deferred what was, as John put it, "mathematical" in their experience to what was "magical"—to what was preternatural or more perfect even than the nature to which scientific law (doled out in weak success rates and scheduled injections) condemned them. Facts fell to feeling: "I always knew it was going to work," John said; "John had a feeling," Rachel confirmed. They recast what might otherwise have seemed the closed world of repro-tech as a wide open fantasy reality: "once you go / through those doors," she said, it's . . . like [there's] no turning back . . . It's, it's, it is the world / of science fiction, Della." Within that mystery theater they performed stories of the many "little mystical things," the omens and remarkable coincidences that surrounded Annie's birth, collapsing what at first seemed easy distinctions between what was natural and what wasn't into a master dub of science fiction, legend, mysticism, superstition, and even the fantasy fulfillment of the ultimate American dream: winning a shopping-spree sweepstakes.

First there was the story of the blue jay. John and Rachel were waiting to see whether the third transfer would work, whether one of the six or seven zygotes returned to Rachel's womb would actually implant in the uterine lining or whether they would be shed with the ripe lining in a wash of menstrual blood:

JOHN: It was a beautiful day in June.
We were just sitting out there, sort of wondering is this
ever going to happen, is it going to work, will it be
this time, will it be next time
What, what . . .

RACHEL: And my period was, well, we had gone through,
this was the third time, and I was waiting for my period,
and, in fact . . . that day
That morning I went up, I was starting to bleed
a little
bit (*swallows hard*).
And my heart just sank. I just said, I just thought . . .
(*voice dropping*)

JOHN: Is that when it happened, it was right at the end of the
cycle?

RACHEL: Yeah. It was when we were waiting for the news.
And my heart just, I just went, "Oh God," "oh God"
(*whispering*): you know, "please, dear God, don't,"
I just, I can't go through this.
And we sat in the backyard and
I was just, I was just, I didn't know what, I was just
praying. Because, you know, . . . you can still be
bleeding and be . . .

And be, you know, have conceived a child, you know,
because it was very light. It wasn't, it hadn't really, it
wasn't really like a *heavy* flow. And I just remember
sitting in the backyard and . . . We watched
    [our cat]
catch and . . . kill a beautiful blue jay.
Which was a lovely sight.
Most pleasant (*sarcastically*).

JOHN: Well, we didn't, no, we didn't watch him catch it. What
we saw, we were sitting out there in the yard

RACHEL: Well, he had it in his mouth.

JOHN: and [the cat] comes prancing into the yard with this
blue jay in his mouth.

RACHEL: Most disgusting thing.

JOHN: Which he does once a year.

DELLA: A jay is a big bird.

RACHEL: Blue jays are big birds, they are, and beautiful,
    and it was just unusual. There was this beautiful
        blue bird, yeah.

JOHN: Here he comes walking into the yard with this bird. It's
so gross. Who wants to see [the cat] with this thing.
We start chasing, trying to get him to drop it. He won't
    drop it.

RACHEL: He won't drop it.

JOHN: Bury it or trash it or something.

RACHEL: The thing is just limp, you know.

JOHN: He just will not, he's shaking it around like this.

And this is just what you want to see at
this moment, anyway, it adds to the sense of, oh
God, here it is. Here's the message from God.

RACHEL: Here's the message from God, this dead, beautiful bird.

JOHN: So it's five
minutes, ten minutes, we're chasing him around the yard.
Trying to get him to drop the damn bird, and he will
not. He's incredibly possessive about it.

RACHEL (*laughing*):
He will not let that thing go.

JOHN: So finally he walks to the front of the yard, and if you
can remember where that sort of . . .

RACHEL: The rhododendron bush is. Right, you know, Al, where,
            you know, where the grill is.
DELLA: Right.
JOHN: And he's just sitting there. Except that he's now let it
            out of his mouth, and it's lying now on the ground, and
                he's just . . . hovering over it.
RACHEL: He's, he's sitting guard. He's a sentinel now, you know,
                he's just guarding it.
JOHN: And we decided, Rachel's just going to make a mad run,
                right at
            [the cat], and try to scare him off, so I can get the bird.
                So we
            position ourselves, we're close enough.

            I scream *bloody murder*, and she comes running right at
            [the cat].
RACHEL: Like a mad woman.
JOHN: [The cat] just . . .
RACHEL: Clapping my hands wildly, screaming at him. [The cat]
                just . . .
JOHN: Finally, just . . .
RACHEL: Takes off. He just looks at me with terror in his
            eyes.
            I went,
            I just freaked out on him.
JOHN: Three seconds later, the bird flies away.
ALAN: Ohhhhh!
DELLA: Ahhhh!
RACHEL: Up to the top, top . . . top, top part of the tree.
ALAN: Great story. Great story (*laughing*).
            You saved the bird.
RACHEL: Yep, yep, and I never got my period.
            When I thought, when I thought I was bleeding.
JOHN: We thought it was dead. It was alive
            (*general laughter*).

That same day, Rachel and John were inside when they heard a strange
sound outside, made stranger yet by coincidence with the jay's phoenixlike
rise from the dead, and more wild and significant yet in Rachel's wild run
on images:

RACHEL: And then the other thing that was, I mean, these were, but Al, these were SO bizarre.
Then, we're sitting out, again, waiting the day of hearing.
We're sitting out in . . . John's study, and we hear this (*blowing sound*).
Bizarre, most bizarre sound we've ever heard over our house, hovering over our house, like a fucking SPACESHIP is over our house.

JOHN (*laughing*):
(*blowing sound*)

RACHEL: We go running out, and who's over our house?
A hot air balloon
(*general laughter*).

RACHEL: He was waving to us (*laughing, oversized*): You know, (*laughing*) saying, "Mazeltov! It's a girl!"
(*laughter*).

I mean, that would do it. That would do it. Doctors in white coats, you know. Jewish doctors in little white coats
in a hot air balloon.

Suddenly the sounds of extraterrestrial transport became a dream-vision of doctors enacting Jewish rites of congratulations, suggesting the ultimate deflation of a panoptical (unseen, all-seeing) gaze: it was "like a fucking SPACESHIP is over our house," she says, a fucking SPACESHIP filled with "Jewish doctors in little white coats." At once oversized and undercut, the image gives Rachel her last guarantee on pregnancy—and suggests exuberant pleasure in what now seems her power to refuse the position of the compliant anatomical subject. Looking back at the "doctors" looking down on her, Rachel seems literally to prick the balloon with hyperbole and parody.[23]

As she did at the tail end of each story, Rachel solicited confirmation of just how bizarre the experience was. "Wouldn't you say, would that be pretty odd if a hot balloon was hovering over your house?" "Yes," I answered then, as I did later when faced with the coincidence of a champagne cork popping as if of its own accord at precisely the moment that John's grandmother (one of a long line of psychics on his mother's side) predicted not only that this third cycle would work but that Rachel would have twins (two eggs did initially implant): "Isn't that a *wild thing?*" We assented each time, to these eccentricities and to John's story of receiving a sign in the form of a butterfly landing on his shoulder and—more bizarre yet—in an age in which everyone wants to and nobody ever seems to win the grand sweepstakes, John and Rachel win the baby store contest John was, in fact, sure they'd win, although not so sure that, at the last moment, he wasn't "praying" that Rachel could hold off pushing until just after midnight, so that their baby would be born on the date selected "at random" by "Uncle Mikie," owner of the area's largest baby superstore. "We had a born winner," Rachel crowed, "we had a born winner, Della, come on." "You guys were lucky, all the way through," I answered. "All the way," Rachel answered in turn. Annie was a miracle by any measure: medical, mathematical, magical, mystical, secular, popular, carnal. In her crowning incarnation she was the queen of the free market, a vision of the consumer finally getting more than she paid for.

As each story wound into or riffed off of the next, Alan and I yielded not only to a multiperspectival reality but to a radically performative one in which the jay rose *as if* from the dead, and the butterfly perched on John's shoulder *as if* his dead uncle and grandfather were answering his call. By underscoring the *as if* here I don't mean to undermine the strength of John and Rachel's claims. To the contrary, I want to suggest, with John Fiske, that "in language the conditional mood (that of the 'as if') is as important as the indicative; it prevents us accepting the indicative as all that there is."[24] John and Rachel perform their difference from a narrowly medical, scientific model of knowledge production. They practice what Fiske calls *localizing knowledge*, producing an alternative reality from the borders of dominant systems, from the margins of imperializing knowledge—for John and Rachel positivist science, for a historian like Carolyn Steedman conventional historiography.[25] Fiske argues:

> The reality produced by localizing knowledge may be quite different from that of imperializing knowledge, but to dismiss it uncritically as "unreal," or "less real," is to participate in imperialization by refusing to recognize not the difference alone, but the validity of the difference. (FISKE 1993:119)

In the intensive, reflexive, cogenerative dynamics of dialogic performance John and Rachel not only recognize different ("odd," "bizarre," "wild") modes of knowledge production but embrace their validity, their respective truth-values, slipping the disciplinary grip of *what is* (what Fiske calls the "tyranny of the indicative") for the greater pleasures of what might be.[26] Performing in the sense of making (not faking) possible realities, John and Rachel claimed narrative space in a place usually dominated by medical science—not by rejecting medical science and the sci-fi wonders of repro-tech but by multiplying their mysteries in other stories, other forms of "proof," other "wild," renegade ways of knowing.

Rachel and John enact the contingencies of narrative knowing. They do not rehearse fixed truths or facts as much as they displace truth into a fantastical, endless, error-driven search for meaning. Ironically, at the very moment of repeating the past, of securing its place in history by reiteration, Rachel suspends its meanings in a highly theatrical present. In the creative act of telling she opens herself and the past as story to the others—spectral, distant, immediate, possible—who inhabit her story, who stretch and press its parameters, answering her even as she answers them. In so doing, she opens the present to the possibility that the present in the past—the immediacy buried in our sense of the past as past and of the present as forever ineluctably slipping into the past—may surge forward into, through, and beyond this particular instance of narrative wit and courage. Threatening an excess of meanings, refusing to be either lost to history or, by the same token, written into official forms of history, John and Rachel's stories take up the challenge of what the performance theorist, Dwight Conquergood, calls narrative knowing:

> Knowledge is not stored in storytelling so much as it is enacted, reconfigured, tested, and engaged by imaginative summonings and interpretive replays of past events in the light of present situations and struggles. Active and emergent, instead of abstract and inert, narrative knowing recalls and recasts experience into meaningful signposts and supports for ongoing action. The recountal is always an encounter, often full of risk. The storyteller struggling for contingent truths— "situated knowledges"—is more exposed and vulnerable than the scientist in pursuit of covering laws and grand theory. (CONQUERGOOD 1993:337; HARAWAY 1991)

Narrative knowing is not something one has but something one does, makes, and feels. It is an elusive, ephemeral property of stories told. As such, it is next-of-kin to *not knowing*, to giving up the security and stolidity of what's already known for the strange pleasures and dangers of the *unknown*.

Discipline ensures that some forms of knowledge and some ways of knowing are preferred and repeated. It is the defensive stratagem in the practice of narrative knowledge. Through discipline, bodies do not so much acquire knowledge as knowledge acquires bodies: discipline yokes action to its own interests and aims.[27]

And yet the institutional resources devoted to disciplinary control (in such apparently divergent forms as educational, penal, religious, and medical systems) reflect both the force it rages against—"wild" and "bizarre" ways of knowing, alternative body politics, sub- and countercultural forms of action—and its own instability. Discipline is tightest where it is most threatened. It is banked highest against a flood. It marks knowledge as always only temporarily dry, secure, orderly, fixed.

In various ways, throughout their stories and our conversation, John and Rachel throw off disciplinary constraints on knowledge. They recover knowledge to their own bodies and to the embodied process of knowledge making. They luxuriate in multiple ways of knowing, alternately hailing the medical miracle of Annie's birth, its statistical uniqueness, their visceral grasp of its meanings (as Rachel would later note, "you feel, you can't, you feel, you just feel"), grandma's psychic powers, John's signature habit of communing with his dead uncles and grandfather, the bloody, archetypal significance of the flying jay, and their practical wisdom in buying from a baby superstore.[28] Ways of knowing proliferate here, each one yielding to, generating, calling up another. Occasionally inconsistent, even incompatible, by the end of the interview they topple in on each other—so that, in the end, John is "praying" for a financial miracle, knowing that if Rachel can put off pushing for a few more hours, until just after midnight— "Would it be so terrible?" he asks (in a Yiddish accent, as if speaking for his entire clan), they'll win the baby superstore sweepstakes.

In telling these stories, in opening and entering these many doors onto Annie's birth, John and Rachel abandon themselves to variety and pleasure in the broad scope of their contact with the world. They simultaneously include and exceed preferences for scientific rationality. They embrace the medical discourses to which they will be ever indebted—and a whole lot more. With each story or part of a story they expand their epistemological territory: they extend the space over which their ways of knowing (each generating others in turn) will have control. In producing and reproducing Annie's birth, they suggest that it is in fact endlessly producible, that it is endlessly, abundantly, irrepressibly, and undecidably meaningful. They enact a world that cannot be fully, finally, causally *explained*—and so cannot be explained *away*. In telling these stories, John and Rachel make present—they re-present—what otherwise tends to disappear under the bright light of scientific theory: the mystery of Annie's birth or the stubborn *absence* of a total explanation. They do not so much reject scientific ways of knowing as they insist on the simultaneous authority of other ways of knowing, with the effect of reducing the authoritarian or absolute value of any one practice.

They refuse to be the subjects of science but subject themselves and their memories to the immediacy of an audience, the demands of time, and the risks of replay—of putting the past into play, of removing it from a place of archival-like safety and letting it change and be changed by the present and future it implies. They thrill to the non- or extradisciplinary force of storytelling. They rewrite authority itself in the language of knowledge as knowing: as a protean, situated, sensual process, awash rather than contained in storytelling.

Refusing scientific mastery, however, they do not refuse linear narrative. To the contrary, they multiply "the possibilities of linear narrative and of 'story,' producing a dizzying accumulation that undermines . . . narrative logic by its very excessiveness" (Suleiman 1990:137). Undermining narrative logic by excess, they produce excess—more and more stories, stories and bits of stories dislodged from linear sequence—suggesting greater possibilities yet. As Mary Russo (1994:181) has observed, "there is always something left over, something as untimely as subjectivity itself, that forms the basis of a new plan, perhaps another flight." Rachel's performance is redolent with free-ranging (excessive) subjectivity. It suggests constant readiness, proximity to something sublime, "perhaps another flight"—the blue jay's, the butterfly's, the ballooning doctors' only promising *more*.

Counterrites

John and Rachel's story is, like most birth stories, about origins. It is about the beginnings of a life and a family. It is about how invigorated death is by birth and birth by death and about how close they are in the soil of life. It is about the renewal of ancestry and the emergence of the mother into maternity. It is a way of securing identity by tracing it to its roots.[29] And it is a hook, a line, into the "original" creation, the creation of creation, the beginning of life itself, reenacted as it is not only in every subsequent birth but in every birth story. It is also highly and variously original—creative, regenerative, even ingenious in its refashioning of birth, in the pressure it puts on the past to yield its meanings, in its abandon to the pleasures of making up the past all over again. In what often seemed the hard necessity of *inventing memory*, John and Rachel mixed origins and originality. The first cause of the story and the act of telling it merged in the sense that telling—and retelling once again—involved founding new origins or establishing new grounds for talk.

Meaning originates where remembering and remaking meet. In the immediacy of the narrative event the narrated event is transformed (Bauman 1986). The past becomes the unstable meaning and origin of a possible/impossible—wild, bizarre?—future. In the perilous process of submitting *knowledge* to *knowing* and *knowing* implicitly to *not-knowing*, even *unknowing*, meaning takes and—just as quickly—changes shape. *Narrative knowing* refigures the world "as a coding trickster with whom we must learn to converse" (Haraway 1991:201). In a trickster world narrative rites can thus unmake and remake the birth rites from which they nonetheless take their license. They can become counterrites. For John and Rachel this meant not only multiplying sci-fi discourses but rewriting techno-sex, criticizing the in vitro process, recovering the body as waste to (re)productive possibilities, perversely asserting the absolute normality of Annie's birth, and projecting fantasy worlds in which none of this would be necessary.

****

The only time my conversation with Rachel became strained was when—over an hour into it—I asked: "Well, tell us what happened . . . with the birth itself?" not realizing that my question had already been answered. My question assumed—conventionally—that birth consisted of labor and delivery. For Rachel, Annie's birth occurred at the moment of conception—or, more specifically, at the moment of fertilization, a procedure, in Rachel's case, isolated from both sex and pregnancy as well as from the common lore of a mighty sperm traveling against gravity and magically finding and anointing its ovular mate. Annie's was a techno-birth—but, as Rachel tells it, no less a birth for that reason. As Rachel describes it, Annie "was born" in a petri dish on their thirteenth anniversary:

RACHEL: On our anniversary.
Fertilization occurred on our anniversary.
DELLA: You're kidding?
RACHEL: No, 'cause that's when it occurred.
That's actually . . .

> It was May 30th, yeah, that it was all fertilized
> and it took place, and then . . . that's when
> it happened.
> And then the transfer was two days later.
> So on our anniversary she was born.

In a matter of seconds Rachel's cool reportorial summary, "Fertilization occurred on our anniversary," becomes "So on our anniversary she was born." Pivoting ever so slightly on the fact that fertilization occured on her wedding anniversary, Rachel rewrites fertilization as birth. This is more than narrative sleight of hand. Especially in the context of all the other "little mystical . . . things" that haunted and supplemented their birth experiences, John and Rachel refuse to understand the coincidence of fertilization and their anniversary as merely accidental. For John and Rachel the coincidence sanctified the event. It gave it—and them—promise and resilience beyond the cold chancy realm of technical procedures. It rooted the entire scene in a personal, family, and human history—a history of weddings, anniversaries, and birthdays, a genealogical history driven by the desire to reproduce itself in future generations: a history, for John and Rachel, as full of the past as of the future, destined, it seems, by cosmic convergence to fulfill itself in a biological child.

In telling stories about it, John and Rachel bring artificial fertilization into the folds of family life. They recover it to the body of their shared history—to the world of feelings, spirit, desire, and complaint, to the ordinary and extraordinary world of relatives, parties, and work in which they live every day. They also make it sexy. In the final analysis, for John and Rachel in vitro was not a wondrous exercise in birth beyond sex. It depended, rather, on what I would call sex by proxy: on the transfer of sexual authority to the med-tech procedure by aligning it with what appears here to be a major event in their sexual life together: their wedding anniversary. By locating Annie's conception in the aura of renewed vows and wedding night romance, they secure its origins in their own sexuality—making the painful, alien, and potentially overwhelming experience of monthly hormone injections, egg withdrawal, and zygote transfer practically incidental to their own baby-making rites.

In returning again and again to the importance of the fertilization/birth occurring on their anniversary, moreover, they rehearse the middle-class heterosexual norms to which their sexuality is at least in part in hoc—including the expectation that once married they will reproduce: they will have children and reenact the nuclear family patterns in which they were raised. In characterizing the anniversary as birthday they thus build an identical foundation for their own and Annie's lives and "normalize" their family relationships: they close the gap between biological reproduction and mechanical production suggested by Rachel's halting substitution—"he knew somehow we were going to / have a baby . . . *produce* a baby of our own"—and remove this strange, new mix of "having" a baby and "producing" a baby into a world of approved social relations.

Slight as this move may seem here, it takes on greater magnitude in the context of Rachel's account of what I wanted to call the "birth itself." In describing the labor and delivery process Rachel further normalizes her experience. She matches it with preset expectations for a birth that is normal in the descriptive sense of being statistically average and in the prescriptive sense of being appropriate: of conforming to *what is* in the name of what it *should* be.

As the social psychologist Carol Tavris has shown, what's normal in and around pregnancy and birth tends to be based on what she calls a "male model": the working assumption in medical practice and scientific research that the white male body is "the prototype of the *human* body" (Tavris 1992:97). On the basis of this assumption whatever is different about (white) women's bodies is a measure of their deficiency. What may be average for women is either "abnormal" in the sense that it deviates from a male norm or "normal" in the sense that it fulfills masculinized expectations for female inferiority and dependency. In other words, "normal" women are "abnormal" men. Through systematic discipline (effected across the "normal" range of punitive wage scales, sexual harassment, sexual violence, the panoptic suspicion of mothers on welfare), women are generally made to feel their exclusion from the regime of white masculinity—from which women of color are typically twice removed.[30] Positioned on the cusp of white privilege, the white women with whom I spoke tended to identify with the codes and practices of white masculinity, to internalize the preferences for masculinity with which they nonetheless struggled, and to punish themselves either for being women or for failing to be like men.

Several of the women with whom I spoke wanted desperately to be if not exactly male then at least macho. They seemed to feel the rewards of normality were so great as to justify sacrificing their difference to norms of masculinity. They punished their female "abnormalities" with exercises in mind-over-body control, as if by mental, rational effort they could even stop being women (leading their male birth coaches to praise them for being "real troopers"). As the literary theorist Judith Fetterly has so suc-cinctly put it, they identified against themselves (Fetterly 1978:xii). A pre-natal instructor chastised herself for having "failed" adequately to manage her labor pain, to fulfill narrative expectations for a controlled birth. In so doing, she felt she'd not only let down the doctors and medical institution to whom she was indebted for professional approbation but had betrayed her students, in whom she had cultivated the same rules for a "normal" passage through birth that she had violated. She'd caught herself in a trans-gressive performance of birth—and punished herself accordingly. A lawyer and mother of three told me—with wistful dismay—the story of another lawyer who, nine months pregnant, had proudly gone without food for the length of a seven-hour deposition. As much as the narrator of this story criticized her colleague's behavior, she still seemed to feel reproached by it for her inability to control the chronic vomiting, dehydration, and exhaus-tion that made her maternal body particularly "grotesque."[31]

Margaret, for instance, found that the only way she could defend her difference from masculinized medical norms was, in effect, to enter into hand-to-hand combat with the medical staff, to fight (masculine) fire with fire. For her second birth (a little over a year before our interview), she had chosen a medical group ostensibly supportive of her hopes for a VBAC—a vaginal birth after cesarean—still a relatively rare phenomenon pursued in the face of medical assumptions that once a cesarean always a cesarean. But, at the hospital, those assumptions reigned with such force that what-ever encouragement Margaret received for a VBAC seemed merely patron-izing or, worse, a setup for failure. Almost immediately, she faced pressure to accept interventions that could eventually lead to, even necessitate, a second cesarean section. As Margaret tells it, the medical staff tried to threaten and to mock her into acquiescence. They used the prospect of "some bad thing" happening to her or to her child to curb her to the norm, to make her yield to their regimen of epistemological control. Given the fact that her first child was lifted from her belly with the umbilical cord wrapped around its neck four or five times, Margaret couldn't simply ignore their attempts to make her do things their way. But, encouraged by her prenatal instructor, she went on the offensive. She insisted—and proved—that she could read her own body better than any monitor could. She outwitted hospital (liability-driven) rationality with practical reason: she not only postponed interventions by repeatedly asking what they were for and why they were needed but made the medical staff defend their appropriateness. And twice she caught her doctors in what can at best be described as misrepresentations—once when "they" tried to convince her that she "just [wasn't] progressing" and once when her doctor denied receiving her baby into this world with his naked hands (supported only by the ultimate instrument of domesticity—a hastily grabbed towel):

MARGARET: so . . . I decided . . . around lunch time that you know
this was probably going to be the day
and I quickly made a tuna fish sandwich because I knew
they weren't going to let me eat anything in the
hospital
and . . . so around three o'clock . . . or four o'clock I said
(*sing-song*): "I think it's time to go" (*Della laughs*).
And we went, and the—nurses were really rude to
me . . . really horrible, rude and nasty.

DELLA: What would they do?

MARGARET: The one, the one that taught—I went to her refresher
class
and the one that taught that was really nice. She said,
"Listen," you know, she said, "I, I have been in those
delivery rooms *so* many times," she said, "*don't* let
them do anything to you, don't let them hook you
up to any monitors 'cause once they do, you're five
steps closer to a C-section," she said, "Just don't do
it," you know, because she knew how much it meant
to me not to want to do that.
So . . . by the time I check in and get to my room . . . a
doc walks in, he says (*very fast*): "You want your
epidural now?"
And I said "I just *got* here!" (*laughs*)
And, so, then this nurse comes and she says well—
I was sitting in one of these—*niiiice* little
rocking chairs

DELLA: Yes . . .

MARGARET: I was sitting in this nice little gliding rocking chair and I
think Stan had
gone to park the car or something and I was by myself
but—and it hurt a lot but it was *fine*, it was just—
being real calm and real centered and not screaming
and not (*laughs over words*), OK.

And so, the nurse says, "You have to get into bed." And
I said, "I don't want to get in bed, I'm perfectly happy
right here." You know, "Leave me alone, I'm fine."
"You *have* to get in bed, you *have* to get in bed, you
have to get flat on your back." I'm like (*sing-song*): "I
don't want to get flat on my back . . ." "Well, we just
have to check a few things."
All right, so—then, you know the—the—this struggle
went on from the—through the *whole* thing, I mean
. . . the baby was born at like, somewhere between
6:30 and 7, so I wasn't even in there for three hours.
And, I would say every ten minutes
they threatened something new
and—said if I *didn't* do it they would give me a
C-section.
So it was horrible
really awful (*laughs*).

DELLA: Well—what was this *threat*ening
about—I mean why . . .

MARGARET: Well it was mostly the nurses and I couldn't understand it
because . . .
the damn belly thing [fetal monitor strap] is not that
intrusive and they could feel a nice little heartbeat
and everything was fine . . .
And so that—that wasn't too bad but then they insisted
on the IV. Because what if they had to give me a C-
section they had to have a line. And then, so then
you're, you're—that— . . . makes your range of
motion—ZERO (*laughs*), you know you can't wander
around, you can't walk, you can't get vertical, you can't
do anything. So, and then they wanted to do
I don't know four or five other things . . . it was
just—um
finally
about the time I was in transition or something, I mean
you know this had been going on a while and I
could tell
. . . well, this was like a Tuesday and the Friday before
I had gone to the doctor

and had the female doctor who was not on call
  this day
and I was, I was four or five centimeters dilated
  on Friday
so by *Tues*day, I knew I was at least halfway there
  on Friday
you know?

DELLA: Right.

MARGARET: And they're saying, "Oh you're not," you know "it's just
not—progressing."

Progressing? I've been here—you know an *hour* (*laughs*).
And it was already bigger than some people—you
know more . . . dilated . . . than . . . when . . . *lots* of
people go to the hospital, you know?

DELLA: Right, right.

MARGARET: Especially someone who hasn't been through real labor
before.

DELLA: Right, *right*.

MARGARET: That was Friday so this is Tuesday. And, so I *knew* . . .
you know . . . something had to have happened in the
meantime . . . a *little* bit
of progression or whatever
so they just kept . . .
harassing me and ummm
then they wanted to start . . .

DELLA: Did you just feel that they just really wanted to do a C-
section?

MARGARET: Yes I did, I did.

DELLA: Were they bothered that you didn't
wouldn't just do this or . . . ?

MARGARET: Well,
the nurse didn't like the way I was breathing. She wanted
me to do it her way. And she like—really made fun
of me, she said (*angry*): "That's not gonna help you."
And it's like, "It is helping me" (*laughs*), you know, "I
feel better when I do it this way" (*laughs*) you know
and . . . she just—I don't know, she was just really nasty.
And finally she got really disgusted and left. I was
happy. And it—it was time for her to go 'cause the

doctor left too—it was a shift change. So—two new nurses came in. They were a little nicer.

But they kept wanting me to *push* and it's like, "I just got here, I've only been here an hour, it's not time to push —

I KNOW." You know, I *didn't* know but I knew.

DELLA: Right, right.

MARGARET: You know, I mean you just know it wasn't time.

And they kept making me push and I was getting really tired from that and there was no *rea*son to, I could tell where the, I mean I could *feel* where the baby was, you know it was like

DELLA: Yeah.

MARGARET: and I could *tell*

it wasn't time.

So then . . .

ahhhh, the doctor came in

and because the baby's head was down, hooked

under, getting ready to go, then they wanted to do

that corkscrew thing [internal fetal monitor] into the scalp and I just had a hissy fit, "No, absolutely not (*both laugh*). Absolutely not." And

then they threatened it *again*, they said, "Well we," you know, "we can't tell if the baby's, we can't hear the heartbeat

so if you don't do this, we're gonna give you a C-section."

And—this is—like maybe I've been in there two hours at this point:

I mean *nothing*! (*laughs*)

You hear about people who were in labor for twenty hours

DELLA: Yeah.

MARGARET: or something so it's like I could understand if I had been there for

a day and a half that they would say,

Let's just go ahead and do this

DELLA: And it wasn't even like

MARGARET: but

DELLA: your first C-section was for some . . .

MARGARET: *No*, for some problem

DELLA: . . . prolonged . . .
             problem. Yeah

MARGARET: yeah like, like narrow pelvis

DELLA: Yeah.

MARGARET: or anything like that. *So*
             . . . the doctor came in again
             and he said, "Well this is gonna take a while," he said,
                 "you're nowhere close to ready," and I said, "I
                 think I *am*."
             Aaaand he said (*very fast*): "No you're not."
             And so he went to like right where the door was and
                 was peeling off his gloves and I said, "The baby's
                 coming
             NOW."
             And he turned around
             and looked
             and the nurses said

             "She's not kidding!" because they can't catch the baby
                 legally
             he has to do it, they said, "She's not kidding!"
             And so he grabbed the towel and caught the baby in
                 the towel.
             And. . .

DELLA: I mean it was that quick (*finger snap*), the baby was out?

MARGARET: Yeah, yeah, oh yeah.

DELLA: just . . .

MARGARET: like, and so, I mean it was real fast
             and so . . . at that point
             everything worked—the pushing, all the stuff that's
                 supposed to happen, all—that they were trying to get
                 me to do before when it—wasn't time to, it worked.
             Then. But it was like before that there was no reason
                 to do it 'cause it was—wasn't *there*, you know?
             And . . . all it did was just make me tired.

DELLA: Which would have been a good excuse for them to do a
             C-section.

MARGARET: Oh yeah (*mock weak voice*): "Oh, she's exhausted . . ."

DELLA: Oh, you're too tired (*both laugh*).

MARGARET: Uh-huh. . . . and,

you know, you wonder how much of what's going on
around you you're aware of when all this is going on
and I said—

about a week afterwards or

sometime—I—I was kinda dreaming about it and

(because I was kinda angry

at, at the way it had turned out) and I said something to
Stan, I said, "Did the, did the doctor

have

gloves on when he caught the baby?" He said, "No."

And so I went in for my checkup, I said, "So, you
know, you—you didn't

even get your gloves on! . . . I *told* you that baby was
going to come." *He* said, " Oh, I haven't caught a
baby bare-handed in five years."

And it was like, I went back home and said, "Stan—

I did see that, didn't I?" You know (*laughing*), this guy is
trying to make me crazy. "Yes, you did see that," he
said, "I was there, I saw that."

And . . .

He really wasn't a lot of help because they kept scaring
him with all the technological stuff, saying you know,
"This isn't going to work out, this isn't going to work
out," you know, you know . . .

and of course he's scared that the baby is not going to
be healthy I'm not going to be healthy

and, you know, I'm screaming at him, you know
(*laughing*): "Don't listen to them, don't let them do
this!" and so

he's kind of in the middle.

DELLA: So you were like

screaming and fighting the whole time?

MARGARET: Well yeah, I mean I had other things to think about

and I'm sitting here saying no to all this stuff that
they're doing, you know, "No, no, no, no."

And fighting—and I'd gain maybe twenty more

        minutes before they'd finally wear me down and
        make me do some
       terrible thing, but
       . . . oh, the other thing I wanted to tell you about the
       the *first* birth
       it may have been
       a good idea, I mean, it may have been a lucky break that
          that happened because when . . . they did the C-sec-
          tion the baby came out bottom first

DELLA: Hmmm.

MARGARET: and, you know, they pulled him out by his bottom and
          the cord was wrapped about four or five times around
          his neck real tightly.

DELLA: Woww.

MARGARET: So had he had to go down
          the birth canal it *may* have caused for—loss of oxygen or
          some bad thing so

DELLA: Right.

MARGARET: You know it's like
          whenever I

feel resentful, I think, "Well, it could've been good."

Unfortunately this fight was exhausting, distracting, embittering. By the end, it is unclear exactly how much Margaret won or lost. Even her last reminder to herself—"whenever I / feel resentful, I think, 'Well it could've been good' "—seems a weak attempt to find a kind of peace available only to those who reconcile themselves with the norm. Someone has to con-cede to the other's way of knowing, someone has to forgive or at least laugh in recognition of the contradictions at work here—and it is clearly not going to be the doctor. Rather than concede, he secures the fort. When posed with Margaret's triumphant account of the facts—"I went in for my checkup, I said, 'So, you know, you—you didn't / even get your gloves on! . . . I *told* you that baby was going to / come' "—he recovers the high ground, rejecting her version of things with a sweeping " 'I haven't caught a baby bare-handed in five years.' " With all the authority of "objective" science behind him he leaves Margaret feeling betrayed, demeaned, and self-doubting. As she put it to herself, "This guy is trying to make me crazy." He doesn't *call* her crazy but succeeds in undermining her confidence enough to *make* her seek reconfirmation from her husband and again, it seemed, from me. He produces her as needy and unreliable—the stereotype of the hysterical woman—even as he reproduces himself as the unwavering professional. How could he get away with this?, I wonder. How could he not only deny but *invade* her story, marking it as his, making her doubt her own authority? How could he so quickly get the better of her? How did he manage to steal away not only her story but that part of her self that took such confidence in it?

For a moment, it seems, Margaret let down her guard. For a moment, fresh with her birthing room victory, she stopped being as defensive as she had to be to gain that triumph. And she got ambushed. She thought the battle was over and found she was sorely mistaken. She was on his territory now, under his spectatorial control. With anger and sympathy, I imagined him surveying her body laid out on the examination table, every part, inside and out, exposed to his critical assessment. Listening to Margaret's story, I watch his obstetrical performance.[32] I catch his quick glance. I see his gloved hands making his instruments and her body practically indistinguishable. I remember with her each laminated tug and push and feel him writing his truth into her body, making her vulnerable to him, making her feel her vulnerability to him, making her *know* herself as he knows her: as the one who is incontrovertibly naked now.

The doctor got to her. He got under her skin, as we say. He confounded her story with the performative power of his own. He exposed it to the same fluorescence by which he examined her body and found both wanting. Performing the role of the professional seer, whose lenses and instruments effectively guarantee his view of things, he reduces Margaret to the size of a manageable specimen. In her role as obstetrical patient she becomes at least in part a display object. The obstetrical patient, not entirely unlike the corpse undergoing the autopsy that Francis Barker describes in *The Tremulous Private Body*, is "expelled from the place of signification to the object status of what is signified." She is made into "dumb flesh"—the body cut off from the mind, incapable of speaking for itself, except as a referent for other people's stories, in this case as the challenging, unruly female that must be recuperated to norms of femininity.[33] She is something between a corpse and a curiosity, more seen than seeing: at once a show of undisciplined sexuality (her orifices gaping, her anger seeping out in "hissy fit[s]") and the spectacular proof of medical supremacy: "The object of a science which in knowing it will master it, and in healing it will accommodate it to labour and docility." If she performs her part well, she will be the "good patient" whose body is a "mechanism which can be understood, repaired, and made to work" (Barker 1984:80). She will be grateful to medical diagnosis for bringing her back into the fold, for recovering her body from both the potential meaninglessness of death and the excessive meanings of deviance.[34]

Margaret's story—and her story of her doctor's story—is doubly ambivalent. As Margaret tells it, she is both divided by and against medical practice. She is "unmanned" by medical authority and self-authorizing in her narration of it. Her story is always already laced with her doctor's (it is marked with self-doubt even as she re-marks upon how "crazy" she felt) but it is also indubitably her story, the right story, the story to which she owns rights (it no more belongs to me than it does to her doctor; you'd better get it right, she seems to demand, not quite trusting that I will but needing at least this rite of witness)—a fact she impresses upon me with stubborn distance even as I verify her account not by objective measures but by absorbing its details in angry anticipation of telling it again; this time, I hope, speaking neither over nor for her but with her, telling what is inevitably my version of her story alongside her own, doubling her voice in mine, mine in hers, strengthening each in turn; in the end, I hope, removing all doubt.

In its doubleness Margaret's story enacts the performative fragility of story: the extent to which any one story is acted on and against another and the extent to which any story thus derives its authority less from an "original" or absolute source (in Margaret's case what "really" happened in the birthing room) than from the control and management of performative resources. How a particular story or truth is performed, how vigorously it is inscribed on and through the bodies of its audience members may be more important to its authority and credibility than its referential value. Thus whether we credit the doctor's story at all, and whether we credit it as fact or story, the difference between it and Margaret's version at least separates truth from his claims to objectivity. It troubles the doctor's authority with the possibility of alternative truths. Even insofar as it directly bothers the doctor only enough to make him more dogmatic in his own point of view, it must suggest to us listening to Margaret that facts may be less fact than figures of force, less a priori referents for truth than powerful weapons in ritual contests over whose truth will win out, whose truth will prevail.

In Rachel's story the lines of contest were not so clearly drawn. On the one hand, as I suggested earlier, she resisted univocality with multiplicity. She did not so much reject what's considered medically normal as embroider it with accounts of paranormal visions and preternatural occurrences. She and John made us see double, hear double, superimposing stories such that each, in relation to others, suggests yet other (dizzying) ways of knowing the body and acting in the world. On the other hand, when it came right down to it, Rachel bounced between two disciplinary models, between two sets of competing norms. When she began to talk about the birth "itself" she traded one kind of normality for another, resisting, it seemed, the compulsive performance of hormonal injections by the equally compulsive reiteration of the classic, normal birth.

As we approached the labor and delivery process Rachel suddenly became more subdued, more deliberate, less given to flights of fancy and passion. Performing the role of prepartum mother to which my question assigned her, she was self-effacing, even willing to let this part of the birth experience disappear under the name of normality. In fact, she initially dismissed the entire birth as "normal" (appropriating to her interests the same story that allowed Margaret's doctor to dismiss her as abnormal) and then—whether because she felt she had to or not—went on to rehearse just how normal it was:

DELLA: Well, tell us, tell us what happened . . . with
    the birth itself?

RACHEL: OK, the birth itself which was . . .

DELLA: 'Cause I never heard your story.
    You held off, you said you weren't going
    to tell me, you weren't going to tell me.

RACHEL: I know. Well, everybody always tells these . . .
    horrible, you know, but it was just, um,
    it was so *normal*. It was just, I think what's so
    great about it, Della, is because the . . .
    the conception itself was so eventful . . .
    That the pregnancy and the birth were so uneventful,
    Thank God, you know, it's like . . .

    So boring, and like a normal pregnancy.
    Just gained weight, had a little bit of nausea, you know.
    Just kind of normal, everything kind of middle of the
    road, no extremes.

ALAN: That's great. That's what you want.

RACHEL: No extremes.

No extremes, Alan, that's it,
just exactly what I wanted.
And she was a little bit early, about, almost two weeks.

JOHN: Ten days.

RACHEL: Ten days early.
And, you know, my wat . . . it was the classic thing,
my water broke.
That was, I felt a little, well, the night before,
I think a lot of women must go
through this, 'cause I've always talked about
this with friends, but . . .
About three days before she was born, I mean,
unbeknownst to me, I was *wildly* nesting.
I was sleeping in her room.
I mean, I just would get up at three in the morning.
(*Everyone laughs*)

ALAN: In the crib (*laughter*).

RACHEL (*joking*):
In the *crib*.
Undoing little presents, you know, packing away things.
Vacuuming upon vacuuming, just getting everything—
But this burst at three o'clock in the morning—*bam*!
Like I'd get up and pee but rather than go back to bed,
I had to go in her room . . . and just (*sigh*)
And I'd lay there and I'd look at the crib,
And it was getting—pow—more passionate, more
    fevered,
within the three-day period,
until finally one morning, at five in the morning,
I went up to pee, and . . . felt this water,
this gush of water come out and a little pink
staining, just like they said, not red but pink.

DELLA: This is textbook!

RACHEL: Textbook classic!

Classic textbook, right.
Water breaks.
What does my husband do?
Go to work (*laughter*).

Rachel wasn't really interested in telling this story. Her telling of it seemed in some ways as perfunctory as the story told. Except for some of the description of "wildly" nesting ("it was getting—pow—more passionate, more fevered"), this exchange lacked Rachel's characteristic hurry and flourish. She summed up the entire pregnancy in one line: "Just gained a little weight, had a little bit of nausea, you know." She counted the events just before delivery in hours and days—as if run now not by hormones but by their prim and disciplined "other," the clock. With metronomic precision she ticked off the timeline of impending events: "ten days early," "the night before," "three days before," "at three in the morning," "at five in the morning."

While she and John had previously staked their confidence in what was "pretty odd," "pretty strange," "odd in the extreme," "odd in the extreme!," Rachel seemed proud of just how lackluster this story was. She insisted on it, repeating, "it was so normal . . . so uneventful . . . so boring . . . no extremes." Recognizing that this was "just exactly what I wanted," she goes on to enjoy how much this story is not her own, how much it fits the medical textbook model (it was "just like they said"), how closely its contents conform to both scientific and cultural norms. In one short vaudevillian take she even characterizes John as so ultranormal that he suits the brute husband stereotype:

> Classic textbook, right.
> Water breaks.
> What does my husband do?
> Go to work (*laughter*).

By (half-joking?) implication, Rachel is "the wife," Harriet to John's Ozzie, nesting, vacuuming, and dropping babies according to plan.

Rachel normalizes her experience in story. By initially dismissing it, even effacing it (presuming it's so normal, so unremarkable, that there's nothing to talk about) and then talking about it largely in terms of schedules and stereotypes, she resists any uniqueness, much less deviance, in her experience. If anything, she covets norms others find oppressive. Rachel submits herself to the "tyranny of the indicative." She constrains her performance to proof of the cultural, social, legal, and medical norms buried in the apparently neutral description of averages, patterns, customary behavior, and routines. She accedes to a discourse of normality that elides *what is* and *what should be*, assimilating her narrative to discourses of normality that not only reify and naturalize certain behavioral models and codes but also authorize the disciplinary maintenance of such codes: they give to cultural and social ideals the look of cool incontestable data and cloak regulatory procedures in "the ways things are around here." In so doing, among other things, she sets one normative experience against another: the delivery against the conception.

For as much as John and Rachel were able to recover some humanity from the in vitro process, especially by shepherding various "bizarre" omens, mystical encounters, and (hetero)sexual associations to their story of it, it remains a scientific and technological ritual that follows and enforces its own set of norms, producing, more often than babies, "infertile" women, women who feel themselves defined by their biological inability to reproduce. As Rachel describes it, the process follows a taut logic of tantalizing hope and despair and more hope through which the mother's body is impressed with its inefficiency and dependency. In the perilous wait to see whether the transferred zygotes "take," to see whether they successfully implant themselves in the uterine lining (almost nine times out of ten a so-called viable pregnancy does not ensue), the prospective mother comes to feel herself a failure and to reject her body as waste:[35]

RACHEL: Honest to God, Della,
            having been through it three times,
            I can totally understand any couple . . .
            saying after one, "Forget it, I can never do this again."
            Because it's so, it's such an emotional,
            you feel, you can't, you feel, you just feel
            like you're going to get pregnant because you're just so
                medically manipulated, and you're just in the hands
                of, you know . . . the doctors and just, your cycle is
                just overtaken by drugs.
            You just, you feel, you naturally feel just *up*.
            It's like being on an incredibly strong cup of coffee
                for an entire month. Like you just (*breathes deeply*) . . .
            And when it doesn't work . . .
DELLA: Somehow this is a function of the doctor,
            the technology and the doctors and just . . .
RACHEL: Everything, going to the hospital.
            You know, you just feel, you're so, you're desperate,

            and you're also positive.

You know, it's a bizarre combination, the juxtaposition
    of . . . feelings, and you just . . .
At least for me, you're *so* high, you're so up,
    you feel it's going to work, and when you
    get your period . . . you want to just throw your
    body in a garbage can.
And *not only* (*louder, gathering momentum*) have you
    gotten your period, and you haven't had your child,
    but you . . .
if you do not have insurance that has paid for this,
you've taken literally about $8,000 and just
flushed it down the toilet.

Which is the *smaller* portion of the pain,
The larger portion being that you . . . are once
    again infertile.

The in vitro process is clearly, as Rachel describes it, a regulatory procedure: a strategic manipulation of desire by which women feel themselves
on the knife's edge of in/fertility. As several recent critics of reproductive
technologies have shown, the procedure is astounding in its capacity to
overcome identity, to reduce a woman's sense of self to a singular, resound-
ing "you . . . are . . . infertile."[36]

Similarly in my conversation with Rachel, I try to pin responsibility for
Rachel's pain on the medical institution. I suggest: "*Somehow this is a function of the doctor, / the technology and the doctors and just . . .*" She agrees and
disagrees. "Everything," she says, and then goes on to describe not what
the hospital does to the prospective mother but the prospective mother's
behavior in "going to the hospital" and her feelings of being "desperate"
and "positive" at the same time. Rachel ascribes agency to the maternal
subject. She reserves for the would-be mother the status of one who *does*
(rather than is simply *done to*), of one who acts on and in the world and
who consequently feels the extraordinary effects of her actions.

It might be argued that this is simply a sign of the system's success in
"blaming the victim"—in isolating women as the architects of their own
marginality and obscuring the extent to which various social and scientific
systems converge on women's identity. But Rachel tells a different story.
First of all, she deindividualizes it. This story is not so much about what
happened to her as it is about what happens to "you" when "you" undergo

in vitro routines. "You" includes Rachel (hence her caveat: "at least for me") but also Rachel as not-Rachel, as the not-I who, for instance, lacks adequate insurance for fertility treatments. When she says "if you do not have insurance that has paid for this, / you've taken literally about $8,000 and just / flushed it down the toilet," she speaks for herself through "others," identifying herself with "any couple" that chooses in vitro. With this narrative gesture she doesn't so much presume on the universality of her own experience as much as she performs the abjection, the potential for the complete desolation of identity in the body-economics of fertility treatments, for wasting the self in identification with financial loss and menstruation as bodily waste. "Literally" flushing away thousands of dollars with that month's eggs, the woman who "fails" in vitro treatments also fails her domestic charge to be frugal and multiply.

But this is only one of several possible selves with whom Rachel identifies in the course of our interview. The performative space of the interview seemed to allow Rachel to slip in and out of selves, to cross subject positions, to work the borders of identities otherwise fixed in rituals or more limited speech contexts—hospital admissions procedures, for instance, or the occasionally competitive rehearsal of birth experiences in prenatal class reunions, or even the talk show/tabloid confession-sensation reiterated in gossip about monstrous (multiple, teenage, postmenopausal, infanticidal, and otherwise illicit) births. Talking on the wide open stage of this interview, Rachel not only took on multiple roles—disidentifying with any *one* role in the process of performing others—but enjoying and cultivating the space that now seemed to emerge *between* roles. Rachel recounted how various rituals converged on her sense of self, apparently producing not one complex self but several, sometimes incommensurable selves. In the process she also traveled among possible selves.[37] She crossed the stages of their production. She moved between and among ritualized identities, articulating and hybridizing their differences, posing one against each other in an identity space, marking/making space for alternative identity formations.[38]

The you in the in vitro story is thus also a critical projection, a carnival refusal of the power of fertility rites to make "you" feel like shit. Rachel's imagery here—"you want to just throw your / body in a garbage can," "you've taken literally about $8,000 and just / flushed it down the toilet"— at once conveys the brutalizing force of the procedure and profanes it with the same surety and confidence with which Rachel laughed in the face of her mother's death. Rachel recognizes, even respects, the power of the in vitro process (almost the way a child thrills to the fairy-tale giant she fears) but makes it subject to her own performance, to her own body in the act of inventing images and metaphors, to the imaginative fertility of story-telling. Exercising her agency as a storyteller, she draws the giant down from the cool and lofty realm of technical procedures to the sensual embodied realm of performance and story and their common (if smellier) correlates in garbage cans and toilets. In her sweeping, unflinching representation of the in vitroed body—the disposable body, the body that mocks the would-be mother with menstrual blood, the body strung out on hope like drugs—she degrades the giant. She refuses his withdrawal into clouds of abstraction and neutrality with the felt evidence of his work: the extraordinary immediate pain of the in vitro process, the alienation of the in vitro "candidate" from her body, and the resulting intensified need to resolve that alienation—to close the gap, to heal the wound, to seal off the leaking body, and quite literally to stop the bleeding—with a baby.

Rachel can clearly afford, on the one hand, to hug the norm and, on the other, to mock its regulatory procedures. Annie's birth was an almost paradigmatically comic one. Not only did it beat all medical odds but it was framed by humor, privilege, comfort, and good health. Where Margaret raged against the medical hierarchy, Rachel enjoyed mutuality. Her delivery experience was no less a ritual than Margaret's—it was no less written over and crossed through with norms, expectations, and social scripts—but its lessons were different. For Rachel her baby's emergence into the world was most remarkable for what it seemed to prove about that world: that it was possible to trust in others without loss, that sincerity and reciprocity can be as real as a newborn's cries and mucous skin. In her doctor Rachel found a talisman of trust. And in the lilting rhythms of her story about the final moments of delivery, she seemed to rub its dusty surface (as if a "big, beautiful" genie might once again appear):

DELLA: You were telling me before
about this nurse that
said, "Push" once . . .

RACHEL: Oh right, the doctor.

DELLA: It was the doctor?

RACHEL: It was the doctor. It was. . .
the one . . . woman obstetrician in
the practice, and ah, I just remember:
We loved her—this big, very beautiful—

she's a big, beautiful woman, heavy, but strong and
very smart, but not . . . beating your
head over with how accomplished she is.
Just a . . . a *worker*, you know, she's a worker.
She happens to be a doctor, and . . . very cool,
    and got
this baby out and just . . . said to me, you know—
finally, it came to the last push,
And she said, "Rachel . . . one more push and she, the
baby's, going to be here."
And they'd sort of been telling me previously, you
    know, keep
going, it's not that much longer,
And it really . . . IS that much longer, and there's a
lot more to go.
But when she finally said to me . . . "one more push."
And I said, "Do you promise me? Do you swear? Do
    you promise me just more push? Are you really being
    honest?"
She said, "I swear to you, just one more push. You
    can do it.
One more push and she's here."
By God! one more push . . . one more push, and the
    baby came
out.

JOHN: Did you believe her?

RACHEL: I did, I *did*, I, I *believed* her.
And I still . . . as I was saying to Della earlier (we talked
    about this),
that *look*— . . . that was such a moment of incredible
trust with someone else that I,
to this day, look for that . . .
tone of voice that she had, to match . . .
the future sincerity of
people, you know, to see, if I can hear that same tone
    again . . . it's like,

I'll buy swamp land in Florida (*laughter*)!

Free Fall

Rachel ends with signature irony, referring the whole bloody mess—death, birth, math, miracle—to a con game, a scam. She knows the game. She's still looking for the *look*, the voice, the confirming, reciprocal maternal gesture, that will take her out of herself and convince her to buy the swamp land in Florida that, even in daring "that same tone" into existence, she knows/we know, she will never buy. For a moment, in "that . . . that tone of voice," she heard an echo of something lost (her mother? her childhood? her self? self-love?) that seemed to fade again into thin air. In this last bit of shtick Rachel sends us rolling in the aisles—but in so doing frustrates the very expectation for satisfying closure she sets up. She bypasses the if-then logic of classical drama and positivist science (if this happens, then that will naturally follow; "if I can hear that same tone . . ." *then* . . . ?) for the now purely fantastical, performative as-if: performing on her doctor's promise (" 'I swear to you, just one more push' "), she calls "future sincerity" down into a possible present only to send it away with a laugh, a joke, a whimsical dismissal, all easily overtaken by a sudden rush to make dinner. It's after ten o'clock. We're all hungry. As if on cue, we exit to the kitchen. That'll be the day, she seems to say.

I wanted the logic to close. I had pressed her to repeat this bit of the story (a version of which I'd heard earlier in the day while we were crossing a street, my kid on my shoulders, hers in the stroller, both of us sweating while looking both ways). I'd asked her to answer my own hopes for a peak, a pinnacle experience that would turn everything else around, that would heal all the betrayals and contradictions she'd recounted and echoed in one grand vision of human connectedness. I wanted to believe in the kind of trust she deserves. But then she goes and turns her back on me, sloughing off my hopes and expectations in a last show of carnival command. With Catskills-like precision, she goes for the punchline: "if I can hear that same tone . . . it's like, / I'll buy swamp land in Florida!" I give up. I surrender to her comic control. And yet I wonder at the joke. Facing that third round of injections, wasn't she, for all intents and purposes, buying the con? Who was more gullible—the new-world immigrant Jew who bought bad real estate on a fast promise (the etymological butt of the joke) or the late-generation, baby boomer Jew who bought into the in vitro world—and, whether by luck or destiny, won? In the end, Rachel outconned the con. I wanted to keep laughing, eat dinner, and go to bed.

* * * *

The meaning of any possible flight lies in part in the very interstices of the narrative, as the many-vectored space of the here and now, rather than a utopian hereafter.

　　　　　　—Mary Russo, *The Female Grotesque: Risk, Excess, Modernity*

Is this autobiography? Biography? Whose? Rachel signs off on Annie's birth in carnival fashion, inscribing it with her inimitable hand, at once claiming it and letting it go into *getting the joke*, landing the irony. Drawn into the pleasures of seeing just what's so funny, and caught up in the pure virtuosity of Rachel's performance, I write this now from within the contours of her story, even as her story shapes mine. I am the enunciative context of her story. I am "I" because I am not her or the "me" of her story. I am not-"me." And yet I am not-not-"me," performing with her in this embodied, unscripted memory play of what was, what might have been, what might be, what isn't, and what is.[39] In the particular intensities of our cogenerative rites, Rachel's/my "I" becomes "we" becomes "you"; each becomes a double self, a performative self, taking the stage that takes us. In an excess of pleasure we laugh at the very im/possibilities of authentic self-expression, imagining ourselves suckered, conned into a bad deal ("it's like, / I'll buy swamp land in Florida!"), and yet performing against the odds. We are doubled on stage, each by the other, each by herself, each by her respective partner, all by others. We are double, we see double: we see the duplicities inherent in language, self, story.[40] We close the show in parody. We perform again the discourses into which we are written—and laugh.

But in laughter, now as throughout, the doors that seemed to close forever behind John and Rachel's decision to pursue in vitro open out—this time to the distant but still distinct possibility of finding that voice, that tone, and yielding to the outstretched arms of her doctor's promise, to complete, trusting identification—eye to eye, tone for tone. In the promise of her doctor's promise Rachel's story seems to resolve for a moment—and yet to tremble there, on the brink of misplaced trust, on the edge of error. With every joke and acrobatic turn of phrase Rachel has cut away her safety net. Rising now to this narrative apogee, she is about to fly—to swing free into what Mary Russo has so aptly called the "aerial sublime": a space of exorbitant, admirable risk figured in the spectacle of the female stunt-flyer (Russo 1994:29). She is so *out there*. She performs this stunt to near perfection, showing with every step in the story show-stopping dexterity, precision, and daring. And yet it is the possibility that she will fall that makes her virtuosity complete, that betrays her precarious balance, and makes my heart beat with desire against disappointment. The absence of a net improves the stunt. It intensifies the risk. It draws life and performance into a knot that could unravel at any second. The slightest misstep would send her into a free fall. There is no con here, no fake reality (oh, for swamp land in Florida). In this performance life is the trick—and Rachel either makes it or she doesn't. From my place in the audience I feel a weird twinge of embarrassment. From some place deep inside that I'd rather forget I'm worried that she will blow the show, that she won't make the perfect turn and swing—and that, free-falling, she will show instead just how weak the powers of the imagination are against the pull of gravity, against the banalities of "swamp land." I hope she will prove my base suspicions wrong. That she will find that perfect tone and achieve that perfect *look*. But she has taught me not to expect too much, not to expect anything, really, beyond the thrill of the show. For a few moments at least, I am glad to sit back and watch, to be the good spectator and suspend disbelief in the illusion that it is she—and not me—who is out there.

CHAPTER THREE

Practicing Pain

WHERE DOES IT HURT? *What kind of pain is it?* Routine questions, as often asked by a doctor or nurse as by a friend who has learned by example and experience standard diagnostic procedure, the first assumes that pain is a primarily physical or physiological phenomenon that is and can be specified to a body part or place. *Inside the ankle. Above the right knee.* The second makes representation a matter of classification. It asks for a type or category.[1] Even in its milder form, *How does it feel?* the second question—positioned as it is after the first—assumes a great distance between the material fact of pain and the representational act of naming or describing it, a distance made greater by referring pain to relatively abstract typologies. *It's a shooting pain. No, more of a burning pain. It's shooting and burning, well, both, no, not exactly* . . . Stumped, stammering, I fall into silence, into what seems the welling chasm between concrete feeling and linguistic abstraction. Pain just can't be named, it seems. It is what it is because it is not language, because it gives the lie to our apparently vain efforts to put feeling into words.

Why then, when I fell off the steps to my back porch, did I also emit such a torrent of words (and nonwords) that my three-year-old daughter didn't know which was more amusing/terrifying—mommy rocking on the ground hugging her right knee or mommy saying all this incredible stuff?

Ohhhhh, shit, fuck this, what a stupid . . . no, no, I'm alright. It's going to BUST, get ice, get ice NOW, I NEED ice, aaagggh, what a fucking stupid thing to do.

Because pain is not necessarily divided against itself in its so-called physical and symbolic dimensions, but our routine practices of pain encourage us to think that it is.[2] And because the ways in which we otherwise, ordinarily name or "do" pain suggests that pain permeates language, refusing isolation to a discrete body part, confusing bodies, feelings, identities, and others, in a complex mess of representation that is inconsistent with diagnostic practice and is fundamentally inefficient. In other words, the extent to which we find or feel that pain can't be named reflects, at least in part, the medicalization of pain and the normalization of pain within a treatment/recovery model.

Within this model pain is the symptomatic expression of the dis/ease medicine is meant to cure. Meaningless in and of itself, it directs the medical practitioner to the point of ignition, the point of illness or the body's failure under stress. Pain is a signal system. It is the effect of neurological transmission that means nothing or, as David Morris points out, means *nothing*.[3] It signifies objective conditions of distress and disease. It marks itself culture free.

Pain thus also becomes symptomatic of conventional distinctions between culture and nature, mind and body, distinctions often crudely deployed in efforts to justify often egregious forms of corporeal discipline, violent knowledge practices, even torture, and to legitimate abandoning women in labor to charges of "hysteria"—that is, of either feeling too much that means nothing or feeling nothing and making much of it.[4] Made to mark—to *sign off* on—nature vs. culture, pain underwrites its own subordination and recuperation to prevailing modes of biomedical knowledge and practice or discourse. Isolated within the body, away from more complex modes of cultural understanding and representation, pain is paradoxically neutral and threatening. It is the shifting line simultaneously dividing and guarding culture from nature.

In this chapter I want to explore the possibility that practicing pain as a primarily physical effect tends to limit and to disguise its cultural implications. I also want to note that, except in some discussions of hysteria and in feminist theory specifically concerned with birth, birth pain is generally elided in discussions of pain that tend, moreover, to think of pain primarily in terms of illness and injury. I consequently want to ask, How is pain represented in birth stories? What is the meaning and significance of its birth story-performance? How is pain *practiced* in and by birth stories? How is it made to mean—and to mean *differently*?

One woman with whom I spoke hoped that this book would not dwell on the pain of giving birth, that it would break with what she took to be the conventional identification of birth with pain. She wanted me to re/present birth, to separate it out from pain and to realign it with more "positive" signs or images. She recognized, it seemed, the power of representation to make birth meaningful and to shape the birth experience. She charged me, in turn, to make *birth* mean or signify differently, suggesting that *birth* was a relatively flexible and contested term, but that *pain* was, to the contrary, relatively fixed. In her admonition to me it seemed that while *birth* could and should be reconfigured within an open system of representation, *pain* was stuck. It meant one thing and one thing only. It was a different kind of sign altogether, linked inextricably, it seemed, to bodily horrors—a link forged, I suspect, in the heat of accumulated "horror stories."

I don't want to dwell on the pain of childbirth or to indulge a conventionally narrow identification of birth with pain as horror or disease. Nor do I wish to suggest that pain isn't painful, that it isn't often horrible, or that horror stories don't serve valuable purposes in their own right, including simply making pain and the meaning of pain the subject of dialogue. But I wonder whether slipping birth away from pain and abandoning pain to discourses of horror and dis/ease doesn't in fact reinforce conventional notions of pain and set women up for terrible disappointment. Pain will inevitably catch up with the birthing body. No amount of representation can hold it off. And when it finds its way into the birthing room, will it be, is it horrible? I want to heed my friend's warning. But, to do so, I think we have to rethink pain, to recite its contingencies within the discourses of birth—and so break not the conventional identification of birth with pain but the identification of birth with conventional notions of pain.

In taking this approach I want first of all to suggest that pain is always at once physical and symbolic.[5] Its meanings are *felt*: they are written into the pregnant or birthing body—by needle pricks, monitor alarms, the slippery caress of IV tubing, a lover's rough grip, a doctor's cool distance, and written by the body—in nausea, tremors, hunger, pleasure, fear, shame. Meaning is immediate in pain although pain is always already mediated by what it has meant, by its past in language, stories, histories, discourse. What pain *is* and what it *means* conjoin in how it *feels*, in the palpable form of its embodied practice. What we know when we feel pain is constituted in the interaction of the self/subject and space, others, objects, often under the numbing, normalizing rubric of routine ("the way things are" or "the ways things are done around here") but also under pressure of an often disguised or displaced specificity. Feeling is particular to the unique conjunction of the feeling self/subject and her material and social conditions in time. It is the flickering trace of meaning inscribed on and by the active, changing, practiced, and practicing body/subject. As such, it remains open, fluid—a complex sign of the eminently unstable relation between the living self and social, structural discourses.

To name pain, then, is to write its history in the sand, to articulate it with ephemeral feelings and sensations. Perhaps because of this ephemerality, because of the evanesence of pain in embodied sign time, pain has often been characterized as prelinguistic. Elaine Scarry, for instance, in her landmark book, *The Body in Pain*, argues that pain exceeds culture and that, in so doing, it not only marks the horizon of cultural experience but threatens to undermine language, identity, culture in all its social and symbolic forms. It holds the peculiar and absolute power to divide us, one from the other, each certain in our respective experiences of pain and yet unable adequately to make that pain understood, each to the other. For Scarry pain is absolute and unshareable. It is "that which cannot be denied and that which cannot be confirmed." It thus has an extraordinary capacity to isolate us from each other and, in effect, from the cultures through whose symbols and stories we find and make common identities.

Pain, as Scarry imagines it, refuses culture. It is not just that pain is hard to express or that, as a culture, we have not adequately cultivated a language of pain. Rather, by its very nature, pain shatters language. It is the agent and means of cultural disintegration: "Physical pain does not simply resist language but actively destroys it, bringing about an immediate reversion to a state anterior to language, to the sounds and cries a human being makes before language is learned" (Scarry 1985:4). For Scarry pain is regressive. It draws us down to an infant or animal feral state that is not only precultural but that, in our culture, tends to be disdained as such. To feel pain, except as a means of its own overcoming, except as a cultivated dare or challenge (especially per the capital credo of the gym and boot camp: "No pain, no gain"), is to yield to nature and incivility. It is to give up *control*—the ultimate sign of a well-managed economy of cultural/bodily meanings.

Scarry's view of pain is conditioned by her primary concern with torture. Torture, for Scarry, "unmakes" the world precisely because it threatens the individual with the total annihilation of meaning and identity. It breaks all sense of cultural affiliation, all access to those bearings by which one identifies as a self in relation to others. I can't disagree with Scarry on the extraordinary impact of pain as torture. Many of the men and women with whom I spoke, moreover, felt they lacked a language for pain and that that lack signified another world altogether, a world not unlike the pre-/postworld Scarry describes, but one shaded with prebirth—with the image/memory of a hazy place where mother and child meet on the verge of life, in the shadow of death, before they enter symbolic discourse, before they are "mother" and "child."[6] These images carry with them an empirical veracity I can't and don't wish to contest.

But I also wonder whether calling pain therefore preverbal or prediscursive, whether decisively locating pain before or beyond language, isn't precipitous, whether it doesn't beg other questions, such as: Where does the practice of calling pain prediscursive come from? Whose interests does practicing pain in this way serve? Could it be that what we experience as an inherent lack in the nature of language is in fact a measure of how far pain has been driven out of language and made to be, to mean its "other"? Finally, then, I wonder whether there isn't good reason at least to entertain (to perform) the possibility that pain doesn't precede language, that it is always already interwoven with meanings and meaning systems. I spoke with one physician who joked about how he could always tell the ethnic background of women in labor by the sounds that filtered through their delivery room doors into the labor ward hallways. Silence apparently meant white, Protestant—and meant that he stopped laughing, or at least so derisively. Could it be that the struggle to name pain is a struggle against discourses that want, as he clearly did, to keep it quiet? Or that value pain precisely for the silence it keeps, for the extent to which, objectified and rationalized in the spirit of post-Enlightenment positivism, it shames feminine/feminist subjectivities, especially under cloak of whiteness?

And if pain is not necessarily outside culture and discourse, where is it? It is hard to find, hard to pin down. It travels. It moves across and between bodies, selves, histories, among feelings and sensations, mapping in its wake a fugitive history, a history of secret meetings and connections. But prevailing discourses of birth pain tend to prefer numbers to networks. They focus either on the length of labor ("twenty-two hours!" "fifty-two hours!") or on the strength and frequency of contractions (measured in minutes, seconds, and monitor signals), or on distinctions between what one prenatal instructor called good and bad pain—pain that was controlled, docile, and "productive" and pain that was wild, excessive, insubordinate, pain that distracted not only from the efficient progress of a scientifically normal birth but from preferences for efficiency and normalcy. These discourses tend to isolate and to regulate pain, to limit it to a physical effect that can and should be properly managed.

But where was the pain in the story I heard that fall day in the Welles- ley grocery store? Was it in the woman's labor, in her body, in the past? Could the physical pain she suffered be in any way separated from her anger, from her sense of injury, from the rest of her life (about which she said and I knew nothing)? Was the pain somewhere between us, in the remonstrance my body offered hers, in what my future held in store? Was it in her pounding, sardonic refrain ("It was a nightmare"; "I'll never have another one") or in her total disregard for my shock, her son's disappear- ance, and the usual protocols of anonymity? Or did it circle and surround us, in our stranger-neighbors' stares, in the false and polite expectation that privilege might keep us all pain free? Pain coursed through the body of that story, that encounter, and my memory along invisible nerveways, keeping me not in horror but in debt and fascination. I carry her pain—where?

In stories. In performance. In the syntax of the body (her body, my body) telling its (joint) history. In the convergence of memory and desire, of the historical body and the imaginary body, on the story told. "Living pain" and language—each crossed through with other stories and histo- ries—cross in the act of re/membering.[7]

In the pages that follow I reflect on some stories of remembered pain. These are not horror stories, nor are they always the same stories that their tellers would tell in the produce section of the grocery store or at a prena- tal class reunion meeting. In general, it seems, explicitly discussing pain in anything but the most conventional terms is beyond the designated scope of everyday birth storytelling. The interview relationship opened another kind of space—one different enough, separate enough, and yet still so resoundingly social as to engage a struggle to name pain, to track its qual- ities and values across birth experiences, sometimes in short, breaking waves, more often in a wash of memory, feeling, and comment.

✳ ✳ ✳ ✳

Karen worked for me. She did for me what she couldn't afford for herself: provided infant and household care for several weeks after the birth of my second child, Isabel, and then cared for Isabel on a part-time, intermittent basis for another seven months. She brought her one-year-old daughter, Jennie, with her, while her husband, Bill, also worked a part-time job and struggled to complete his undergraduate degree.

Karen was in her early twenties—twenty-one or twenty-two—at the time of our interview-conversation, and feeling the first flush of her second pregnancy. As the pregnancy began to wear on Karen, so did Jennie. Jennie stopped sleeping through the night. She became increasingly demanding and anxious—and nursed relentlessly. The dark circles under Karen's eyes deepened. She began to walk with a heaviness I'd never seen before, turning her head slightly away to talk, apparently to hide the rash that had overtaken her usually clear, white-olive skin. She seemed to grieve now for the days she spent painting before she met Bill—days she described to me while we sat together at the bottom of the hall stairs, waiting for Bill to arrive to take her and Jennie home. She seemed to slip into another body as she talked, a body longing for creative expression, a body fueled now by a kind and degree of desire I thought I understood until I visited her apartment months later and saw the huge, raging canvasses that covered its cinder block walls. The paintings frightened me. They were nightmarish, even hellish, in their sweeping dark browns and reds.

Why had she stopped painting, I had asked. Why didn't she take it up again? Bill had insisted she quit, she explained, patronizing my ignorance: because she would become so obsessed with her work that she would forget her other obligations, because she would end up covered in paint—her face, her hair, her clothes—exposing herself and her kids to toxic levels of lead. She had even—once or twice—woken from a spell of creativity to find herself eating paint—licking her skin and pallette, unconsciously satisfying the hunger she'd failed to notice with the very medium of its expression, suggesting something both animal-like and autoerotic. She couldn't risk, as Bill often reminded her, contaminating her breast milk in that way again.

It was at such moments that I felt most keenly the inequities in my relationship with Karen—and yet in ways that didn't always favor my position as the boss, the employer. I envied the depth and strength of Karen's desire. My household needs—the dishes and meals and laundry—and the work for which I left Isabel in Karen's care (delayed writing, committee and course work) seemed paltry by comparison. I wanted for Karen and for myself through Karen what, however nostalgically or romantically, she wanted: a world of expressive desire in which she not only happily but dangerously, erotically lost herself. My desire poured into hers; hers spilled into mine. Together we imagined what we could imagine, perhaps only because it was imaginary, because it was impossible: a world in which the demands of Karen's children, husband, boss, my children, and my body on Karen dissolved in a rough swirl of forbidden paint.

My mother's generosity in paying for Karen's services, moreover, reminded me of the literal and emotional distance it was meant to cover and indebted me to what amounted to Karen's surrogate mothering. In fact—almost fifteen years younger than I was at the time—Karen was my ideal mother: she performed the most intimate tasks for me with ceremony and tact, she gave me and my family the unstinting care she deserved herself, and she loved Isabel intensely.

Karen was, moreover, paid pretty well. More than once she'd teased me with reports of what her family back home in the mountains of North Carolina or friends in the married student complex where she now lived would say when she told them about her job and wages: " 'You get paid *that* for *that*?' " she'd laugh. She took mocking pleasure in the flexible hours and the chance to bring Jennie along, and joked about the strange economy to which we, each in our own way, were bound. In these brief moments we were daughters and mothers together, loosed into a reflexive awkward trust by a distant payroll. But we still often felt guilty toward each other: I for never being able to pay her enough, she for getting as much as she did.

And then there was the problem of Isabel. Soon after our interview Karen decided that she not only had to quit working for us but that she had to quit this line of work altogether. She was dreaming about Isabel. About birthing her own baby and "it was Isabel." She had apparently taken Isabel in like paint, giving herself entirely over to what pleasures there were in this work, giving both Isabel and me great joy and yet, at the same time, finding in the passion she devoted to our joy great danger. When she told me, "it was Isabel," Karen seemed afraid. Her eyes darted behind the pregnancy mask that now covered her face. She continued to fill the dishwasher that day, continued to visit after she left and occasionally to write after she moved away, but the break was clear and, as I only began to understand months later, necessary. To the very extent that differences between us had begun to break down, Isabel and I had to be put aside.

We came to our conversation about Jennie's birth, and Nat and Isabel's births, from opposite ends of the house: Karen had come into the kitchen from the den where Jennie was sleeping to warm a bottle for Isabel; I came in from my study to ask her what she thought about the "husband-coached" model of childbirth—an issue I was trying to address in the preparation of this book's introduction. She responded with her usual ascerbic wit—"It's not all it's cracked up to be"—and then was halfway through a vivid account of her own birth experience before I thought to record it. I fumbled for permission and eventually resumed my place at the kitchen counter, recorder in hand—while Karen remained standing on the other side at the center of the center of my house, managing the stove, the drawers and cabinets, the bottles, and the mess of plates, crumbs, and formula that surrounded her, continuing to rock and to tend Isabel who rested on one hip and against the smooth, taut muscle of Karen's upper arm as if she were where she was always meant to be.

Here, in this strange, midday mid-zone, our roles were multiple and complex. Boss and employee, mother and caregiver, friends, mothers, daughters, mothers of daughters: Karen cared for my baby; I listened out for hers; we passed Isabel back and forth between us as we did the subject of the conversation. The conversation eventually wrapped itself around both of us, as Karen asked me about my second birth and we began to trade birth stats and tales of back labor with the speed of kids playing slap jack:

KAREN: Were you . . . more . . .
were you stronger? for her—
like not letting them bully you around and . . . ?

DELLA: Well . . .

KAREN: I mean like did you think that . . .

DELLA: . . . sort of, it was . . . but the birth itself was more . . .
was so disorienting because it was SO fast,
I mean Karen mine was so much faster than yours
because I was

KAREN: Wow!

DELLA: I had preterm labor

KAREN: Oh . . .

DELLA: I was in bed for ten days. So I was
fully three centimeters dilated

KAREN: I was six centimeters when I got

DELLA: Well see I was three centimeters before

KAREN: before . . .

DELLA: labor

KAREN: even started

DELLA: I was like seven centimeters when I got to the hospital . . .

KAREN: Oh my GOD!

DELLA: In the car *from here to the hospital I went from*

KAREN: Wow . . .

DELLA: contractions eight minutes apart to two minutes apart—
or less than that by the time I got to the, to the *floor*
they were, they were on top of each other.
And . . .

KAREN: Wowww . . .

DELLA: And it was like an hour and a half
from the time I got in the room
to the birth, and it—
well I don't know how it was! I opened up like five
centimeters in the last half hour, or something
like that.

KAREN: (*laughing*):
Wha . . .!

DELLA: And
so it was really crazy and it was all very intense back
pain so and it was really crazy pain too. And it was
just, I was just so much not expecting . . .
I had gone through this *long* negotiation with my
obstetrician about how . . . about this birth plan and he
had supposedly sent it to the hospital because I knew
that it was going to be really fast and I wanted to
really specify things like, like low light.
So you know, I thought that keeping the lights low
was just a *basic thing*
and . . . they kept . . . every time the nurse *left the room*
she would turn the lights on.

KAREN: (*laughing*):
Oohhh no!

DELLA: and then Alan would go run over there and turn them
off and then she would come in and turn them on.
And then, umm

KAREN: Did you ever find the—
could you talk through any of this?

DELLA: No—see—I was so—

KAREN: 'Cause you were so busy . . .

DELLA: —almost immediately just in such incredible pain

KAREN: Gosh!

DELLA: and I also was—to relieve the back pain—I was always
curled over in bed

KAREN: Me too.

DELLA: so I couldn't *see* anybody, and nobody took any pains to talk to me

KAREN: Yeah

DELLA: or move so I could see them
and . . . and the doctor was really weird and the nurse wouldn't . . . she kept
resisting us—we kept saying you've got to call the doctor right away, I said, "Have you called the doctor?"
(*patronizing tone*) "Well, no, we'll
wait and see." I'm like, no, you don't understand this: the birth plan specifies
it's gonna be very fast, it *was* very fast and she'd say
"Well we'll wait and see till you're ready," you know, because they would not believe anything that we said

KAREN: right.
That's *awful* . . .
I got a lot more respect than you did.[8]

We were supposed to be off in our separate corners, doing our separate jobs. But, as the conversation proceeded, and as Isabel became the token of its passage—passed from one set of arms to another, back and forth, across the counter between us, as I interviewed Karen and she reciprocally interviewed me—it became clear that those jobs weren't entirely separate. They couldn't be separated out from the work of each other's body. Our bodies, interests, were twisted, entangled, one in the other.[9] Karen cared for my baby; I wanted to know about birthing hers; she wanted to know about birthing mine; I controlled much of Karen's time; she challenged the very class structure in which we both labored—to talk, to give birth, to make a living, to live with maternal and competing sexual, creative desires.

The kitchen—conventionally understood as a domestic space, a "separate sphere" of women's work and lore—was suddenly a public intersection where our bodies and work, our most personal and our most public lives, crossed.[10] Whether because we met in the course of our respective work or because my initial question about husband-coached birth set a reflective tone or because the appearance of the tape recorder seemed suddenly to throw open the door to anyone who wanted to listen in, the interview soon became an exercise in navigating such public/private crossways: in making privatized pain public and correlating it, in the end, with public funding structures.

* * * *

The story Karen told me or, rather, the story I remember Karen telling me—the story reconstituted within the body of my own (narrative) experience and through the shifting mix of our respective, remembering voices (represented here by a blend of italicized narration and direct quotation)—began something like this:

It was 11, 11:30. Karen woke up to jabbing pains in her lower back. The contractions were coming fast and hard. She woke Bill. How long could she hold out, he asked. Maybe two hours. And that was it, "that was it!" *He proceeded to pile up two hours worth of laundry—clothes, sheets, the comforter off the bed—and to wash and hang every last piece. He drew it out, lingering inside a little while longer, fussing over the proper way to hang the comforter, keeping Karen to a two-hour contract. Karen would plead, saying, You know, Bill, it's getting really bad, I need to lean on you, I can't take anymore and he would say,* "'I gotta get this laundry done!'" *trying to hold off going to the hospital for as long as possible. Karen started pacing outside, working her breathing, hunkering over contractions that were coming faster and harder, bearing the nervous giggles of two men hanging out* "talking about something, sports or something" *in the dark.*

"And then, and then he kept putting me off because he had to do this comforter, which was ridiculous and I just walked. I just, I just stood by the car debating whether I should get in the car or walk. So I walked and, and uh, cause I thought if I get in the car I'm gonna waste so much time waiting on him and then he is gonna not drive me there. He is gonna insist, and then I'll have to argue with him and that might take five minutes and I don't have five minutes, so I started walking."

Bill caught up, carrying the hospital bag, just as Karen was passing out of sight, crossing over the main road to the hospital. She could see the hospital entrance just ahead—it was maybe two blocks away—but could take only ten, fifteen steps before she had to stop and lean into Bill, "and have my contraction"; *ten, twelve steps, contraction, contracting,* "it hurt in my back" . . . *a few more steps, and finally the campus police officer who tickets the parking lot picked them up and carried them to the emergency room. They got a ride part way there—*"and it still took a half hour!"

How did you do it? I had to ask. How did you endure waiting, wading through the pain? "I play, I imagine . . . I got into this deep thing where I was, I was running a race and I could see the finishing line and the other way was the coast . . ."

The undertow kicked in when Karen arrived at the hospital and felt herself suddenly subject to a vast, impersonal "they":

KAREN: The bad part was just laying down

DELLA: When you finally got to the hospital?

KAREN: in an examination room.

DELLA: So they told you you had to have an IV and you had to . . .

KAREN: They just stuck it in
   my hand
   and I said, "I don't need this."
   She said, "I can tell you are strong as a horse but we have
    to, it's regulation"
   "it's policy," they said
   they used one of those words but I knew it was because
    they were liable or something. Well,
   later I knew.

DELLA: And they had to put the monitor on you too? They said
   they had to too?

KAREN: They took it off (*baby cries*), they took it off though, she
   was coming so fast and I had asked to have it off.
   And I was like (*laughing*), "I really need this off" (*laughs*).

DELLA: Cause you just wanted to move or . . .

KAREN: Uhhmm. I wanted to—
   they had me on my side I don't know it was just the
   wrong kind of pressure and it just wasn't, didn't feel
   right.

DELLA: They had you on your side not on your back?

KAREN: They let me lay on my side . . .

DELLA: Because you asked for it . . .

KAREN: They told me to.

DELLA: They told you to?

KAREN: Told me.

Held to shore by a nurse who "got right in my face / and talked loudly so that it was like she was talking / over my pain / or like she had been there or . . . / so I could hear, even though I felt like I was drowning," Karen pushed through to the "good part." Jennie arrived just over an hour after they finally made it to the hospital—to a chorus of shouts and laughter, and blood and water splattering the doctor's glasses:

  . . . towards the end
  they said, OK the baby's almost here, and I looked at

> Bill and I was like AAAAYeeeaaaah and we're both:
> Yeeeeaaaah (*both laugh*)!!
> I said I can do *this* again *real* soon! (*Della laughs*)
> We were already talking about the next one like oh . . .
> that was *neat* to have a baby (*both laugh*)
> we were making jokes about, you know . . .
> I mean the contractions were coming real close together
>> I mean I think she was about to be born but we at
>> least smiled at each other and then as *soon* as she was
>> born I know we made comments and jokes about it,
> about how easy it was (*laughs*).

Karen quickly assimilated Jennie's birth to the scale of relative ease/difficulty she had developed in earlier conversations with new and expectant mothers. "Mine was the easiest," she admitted, a smile just breaking at the edges of her mouth:

> The pain I've heard about was not as bad as mine, I mean,
>> was worse than mine; mine was not as bad as theirs
> it didn't hurt to *me*
>
> I felt *really* lucky
> I felt like I got out easy. . . .
> It was a bad pain but it wasn't nearly as bad as I could
>> imagine
>
> it was much better than I thought it would be
>
> I'm really lucky, I'm really lucky.

Karen not only understood her birth in comparison with other stories she'd heard but as fundamentally like the other experiences she knew only as stories, in other words: as itself a story unfolding, writing itself even as she read it, paging through each of what emerged as the bad, good, and worst parts to the end. The stories she heard, hoarded, cultivated prefigured her experience by their very status as stories, positioning her self as the subject of a story always already (being) written. Her experience was, in many ways, foretold, fore-storied—not in precise detail, not in the sense of story as prophecy, but in its felt forms and expectations and in the options (or lack thereof) she consequently felt lay before her.

Unlike many of the women with whom I spoke, Karen had heard a lot about the pain of childbirth before she gave birth. In her experience pain was not taboo, not forgotten to language. It was, rather, hailed by stories told in and around the university's married student complex, taught in prenatal classes, and shared with her by her mother. Karen had tried to "prepare" herself for the pain of childbirth. She went into the birth process carrying with her a host of interpretive frameworks—stories of an accidental homebirth, of her mother's labor migraines, of women fighting off medical interventions, stories that encouraged her not to be a "wimp," to "breathe through the hard parts," and to look forward to the "gift" that would finally make what she imagined was "the worst pain you can have" seem worth it:

KAREN: It wasn't as bad as other people's labor.

DELLA: What did you hear? you heard stories of other people
and it was much different ?

KAREN: Yeeaah. Yeah. Like the when they don't make progress
and they just get
the pain and then there's no
no
dilation or whatever . . . you know . . . so
I didn't get that. Everything just
went . . .

DELLA: Had you heard lots of—I mean living at [the married
students' complex], does everybody tell you . . . ?

KAREN: Yeah, we compared. Mine was the easiest.

DELLA: Really?

KAREN: Of anything. Yeah.

DELLA: What were some of the good ones, did you hear good
ones?

KAREN: Yeah, I heard some about one couple that didn't make it
to the hospital.

DELLA: *Really?*

KAREN: Hers actually must have been a lot easier than mine
(*laughs*).

DELLA: Was that the one in your [prenatal class]?

KAREN: Charlotte.

DELLA: Charlotte, yeah that's right (*Karen laughs*).
Yeah, well she was
she was
unbelievable.

KAREN: I mean I could've not made it too because

DELLA: Yep

KAREN: If Bill had insisted that [I stay home longer]—well no, I
               knew, I knew it was time to go in
            he just . . .
            but . . . she didn't even *know*

DELLA: She just kept fighting it, I mean,
            not *fighting* it really, but just

KAREN: Putting it off

DELLA: Yeah, it was like "I'm not going to be wimpy" (*both
               laugh*).

KAREN: Yeah, I didn't want to be wimpy . . .
            but I really, I really thought it was going to be a lot worse.
            Because all this time I've been imagining (*whispers*) the
               worst *possible pain* (*laughs*) you can imagine—
            this wasn't that . . . for me.

DELLA: From your prenatal class—I mean, where did you
               get that?

KAREN: Yeah, from

DELLA: . . . from instructors

KAREN: Lamaze.

            See, [the instructor] wanted to *prepare* us
            and not say, you know: you can get drugs to cover it up
               or you can do this or that
            and get out of it.
            This was telling us how to breathe through the
            hard parts, and we'd seen films
            and I couldn't imagine seeing—having something that
            size come out and
            not
            not be the *worst* pain you can ever ever feel. My mama
               told me.

DELLA: Really?

KAREN: Yeah.

DELLA: Had she had—she—had natural childbirth?

KAREN: Ummmm, I think she did with my brother, she had a—
               ummm—
            spinal
            block

DELLA: Spinal block?

KAREN: with me.

              Mm-hmm.

DELLA: So she said with your brother, it was this incredible
              pain?

KAREN: She said it was painful
              with me too.

DELLA: Oh yeah?

KAREN: She said it's like the worst pain you can have but then
              it's all over
              it doesn't last that long and then you have this gift
              so

DELLA: Hmm ... hmm ...

KAREN: But I, I felt *really* lucky
              I felt like I got out easy (*both laugh softly*)
              You know?
              I did.
              It was a *bad* pain but it wasn't nearly as bad as I could
              imagine.

The stories Karen heard prior to her own birth experience structured her experience. They gave her a way to think about and to perform her pain. They interpolated her by fear and desire into specified narrative roles, enrolling her in the drama of beating or bearing the physical anguish that they also promised.

But, more important perhaps, they pointed her toward what would follow the pain. They positioned pain within a story, within a process of moving with some version of heroic strength, feminine grace, or human necessity from a beginning through a middle to an end. They subordinated pain to familiar and predictable patterns of action and outcome. They displaced pain into sequential structures of causality (this happened because of that), chronology (first this, then that), and risk assessment (this will or won't be worth that), effectively diminishing the power of pain in "real" life by cultivating its place in story.

In other words, birth stories critically function *as stories* in the project of controlling birth pain. Their "story-ness" is at least as important as the particular recommendations they make. As stories, birth stories encourage expectant mothers to think *in* story, to anticipate an end, to yoke what will happen to what has happened—in effect, to *tell* the future: to make forthcoming events conform to stories already told. They give women and men a structure to hang on to, a craft on which to ride what Karen would call unintelligible "waves" of pain. Although we tend to think about stories as constructions after the fact, as retrospective accounts and analyses (events must be over, it seems, before a story can begin), birth stories are, in fact, as often imaginative preconstructions as they are reconstructions of events. They are written into the very "experience" we later narrate.

By the same token, they overwrite that experience with prevailing expectations for birth, limiting the possibilities for telling pain to the ways in which it has been conventionally known and told. In the context of the stories Karen heard, moreover, the "power of knowledge" was, as she noted, "power over [pain]." The more she knew, the more stories she heard, the more fully equipped she felt to address what she also knew and learned through stories: that pain would be her adversary in scenes of trial and contest. Pain was the object and test of her subjective control. Even the stories taught in her prenatal class (by a nurse who had been banned from hospital instruction because the stories she told and the narrative positions they offered women often contradicted those favored by hospital routines) divided her self against her pain, drawing her into identification with either the "wimp" or the "bully," the playground whipping boy or the brat, both masculine figures, both configured within a model of pain as power inflicted or suffered, pain as assault or injury.

I appreciated the stories circulating through and around Karen's story. I also realized that the questions I put to her favored the storyness of story, that they complied with the rule of plot and action sequence by focusing on *what happened*. I wanted to know what happened. But I also wanted to know what didn't. I wanted to know what there was behind this rock, this dumb, puny-faced good/bad/worse "pain" that seemed to stand between me and Karen and to taunt my desire to know more or something else or *otherwise*. Adjectivally *easy* and *bad*, pain repeated itself throughout our conversation like the dull throb of an oncoming headache, obscuring far more than it revealed. Equally frustrated by what seemed the comparative cap on Karen's story/pain and by the narrative insurance I seemed to be offering her and others before her, I found myself asking the simple question that I had, nonetheless, yet to ask anyone else: "*What was it like? I mean can you . . .*"—and was suddenly awash in her reply:

Pressure and
stretching and
breaking

splitting open and it was coming out my anus and
you know just
shheww (*slicing the air in front of her*)
(*laughs*) all the way through your whole body
the biggest pressure and
deep pain like
waves and then I felt like I was kinda under and seeing
   these stars and what happened was I was pushing so
   hard at the end I was busting blood vessels in my face
so I was just pushing too hard and I had
you know
my eyes closed real tightly.
Pushing was kind of a relief because that was when
ahhhhh my water finally broke and
wwoooshhhh . . .

This was an extraordinarily performative moment—one in which the narrative itself seemed to split open and to give way to Karen's embodied memory, a memory that now overtook her body with pleasure and pain. Karen was instantly, visibly sweating. She looked away from me, turned away from me, her outstretched arm and arrow-firm hand now slicing the air in front of her, clearing a path from head to groin, again and again, tracking pain's course and welcoming it in. She reached for a glass of water. Explained that her performance—her embodied recollection of what it was like *then, now*—made her feel "anxious and excited." In the doubled im/mediacy of remembering pain, of recalling its particular feelings and sensations in the act of telling, Karen seemed to know a kind and degree of pain relieved of its schoolyard/wartime identification with injury, assault, annihilation. Here, in this antechamber not of language per se but of given narrative forms, Karen's pain rose up to meet desire (her desire? my desire?) in an excess of pleasure, in more desire, in pleasure that exceeded itself in power—not power over pain but power to perform pain, to name it in image and action, to insist in language on the absolute integrity of body, memory, and subjectivity, and to become herself, to enter becoming, in the *act* of remembering pain.

Listening to and watching Karen, I knew the pleasure Scarry felt when she described her own experience of hearing pain spoken, performed, not as the object of control but as the subjective pool of identity itself:

Though the total number of words may be meager, though they may be hurled into the air unattached to any framing sentence, something can be learned from these verbal fragments not only about pain but about the human capacity for word-making. To witness the moment when pain causes a reversion to the pre-language of cries and groans is to witness the destruction of language; but conversely, to be present when a person moves up out of that pre-language and projects the facts of sentience into speech is almost to have been permitted to be present at the birth of language itself. (SCARRY 1985:6)

But while I concur wholeheartedly with the felt sense of Scarry's image, it simply isn't the case that Karen moved up out of "pre-language" and projected "the facts of sentience into speech." What was so remarkable about Karen's performance was its divergence from what was already spoken or reined in by language, its refiguring of given syntaxes, narrative forms, and tropes. Karen didn't just name pain; she re-marked it. She took hold of language, stole, broke, and played with bits of cast-off words and phrases, turning, if only for a moment, the grand story that makes it possible for us even to conceive of something like the "birth of language" inside out.

Scarry echoes the founding mythos of Western Judeo-Christian tradition. To suggest, as Scarry does, that to name pain is to initiate the birth or rebirth of language is to reiterate, at least in part, Judeo-Christian creation myths in which the word divides chaos and form, making chaos meaningful in form. Scarry tells and Karen rewrites a story indebted to habits of difference born with the mythical genesis of the Judeo-Christian world, by which God *named* light and light emerged from darkness and day from night. The world as we know it was in effect born in language and, through language, in *division*. Naming was sorting. To call light *light* was to distinguish it from darkness. It was to introduce into chaos and confusion codes of difference and distinction by which we know that this is this because it is not that. With names come distinctions, and, to the extent that some forms of distinction are prized above others, so too are some names. Difference follows from naming like the placenta from a mother's womb—it is the second birth, the after-pain that is nonetheless the slippery foundation of our very sense of identity and being in the world.

In the Judeo-Christian story of Genesis, moreover, Adam performs God's role on earth. He is the human purveyor of the word. By naming the animals and plants in Eden, by sorting them out by species and genus, class and type, he redeems them from chaos and fulfills the promise of creation. Through linguistic differentiation he confers on the animals and on the world in which they live identity and order. Just as parents do when they name their new babies (selecting the name by which they will be distinguished), Adam carries the animals in Eden over the last threshold of nothingness into being.

The main Judeo-Christian creation tale thus links creation and language (and language with difference) and gives the prerogative for both to men. Whether we are talking about organic life or words, men traditionally bear the first and final responsibility for their delivery. And what is then written into the Western notion of creation (again, whether we are talking about words or lives) is division, difference, and separation—the very means and terms of pain: rending, splitting, "stretching and breaking," the rupture of the mother's body in birth, the separation of the child's flesh from the mother's (a pain with which Kristeva says a mother is "always branded"), even Karen's separation from Isabel or her withdrawal from the seductions of paint and canvas *in the name of* birthing her own child.[11] Within Western tradition creation is pain. It entails not so much making something out of nothing as it does making one thing into two—and articulating, even enforcing a gap between the emergent forms.

How are women themselves written into this tradition? How does the story name them? According to the Victorian and Puritan interpretations in whose shadow we are, to some extent, still living, woman is the linguistic residue of man. She is man's other or not man—the negation by which he secures his own identity. Born of man—like Eve from Adam's rib or Athena from Zeus's head—she is nonetheless man's *difference*, what he is not, the other that defines the one.[12] She is man's inside turned out, banished to the margins of significance and to the edges of masculine control. As the big story goes, she is not only the temptation that draws him away from a natural state of grace but is, to the contrary, the very image of dependence and connectedness—of sensual, carnal *in*distinction—he lives to break. Accordingly, the pain of childbirth is both the "curse" she must suffer for eating the apple in the first place and a reminder of the wanton chaos from which his words must save her.

For a few moments Karen threw off the oppositional (adamic) model of birth storytelling and named herself and her body in her own terms. As if reclaiming a birthright, she spoke as Eve might have spoken had she not been spoken for, had she been able, in effect, to get a word in edgewise.

Ursula Le Guin imagines such an Eve. In her short story "She Unnames Them" Eve uses her husband's gift of speech to "unname" the animals. Using words to undo words, she relieves the world of opposition, difference, and distinction. In the resulting namelessness any one thing threatens at any moment to become its double. Sensuality reigns. Eve describes the resulting erotic confusion:

> None were left now to unname, and yet how close I felt to them when I saw one of them swim or fly or trot or crawl across my way or over my skin, or stalk me in the night, or go along beside me for a while in the day. They seemed far closer than when their names had stood between myself and them like a clear barrier: so close that my fear of them and their fear of me became one same fear. And the attraction that many of us felt, the desire to smell one another's smells, feel or rub or caress one another's scales or skin or feathers or fur, taste one another's blood or flesh, keep one another warm—that attraction was now all one with the fear, and the hunter could not be told from the hunted, nor the eater from the food.

LeGuin's Eve subjects herself to her own rule and leaves Adam's house for the unnamed world. But rather than abandon herself to namelessness, she demands of herself a new language, a way of speaking commensurate with the very act of *walking out*. "I could not chatter away as I used to do, taking it all for granted," she says: "my words must be as slow, as new, as single, as tentative as the steps I took going down the path away from the house, between the dark-branched, tall dancers motionless against the winter shining" (LeGuin 1985).[13]

Karen similarly walked out on discourse, founding in her performance a politically insurgent poetics of maternity, femininity, and birth that was mixed, multiple, inclusive. Rather than choosing one way of speaking or another, she combined multiple ways of knowing and speaking, joining image ("pressure, and / stretching, and / breaking"), commonplace/cliché ("I was kinda under and seeing these stars"), narrative ("and what happened was . . . "), analysis ("I was pushing too hard and I had / you know / my eyes closed real tightly"), and interpretive reflection ("the biggest pressure / and deep pain like / waves") into a single expanding phrase. She slipped back and forth from the grand to the banal and back again, passing from high irony ("deep pain like / waves") to sound imagery ("wwoooshhhh"), from a spilling, material, grotesque body ("it was coming out my anus and / you know just / shheww (*slicing the air in front of her*) all the way through your whole body") to sublime inspiration ("seeing these stars"), back to the grotesque everyday world again ("I was busting blood vessels in my face").

She at once spoke her body and her body spoke her, simultaneously articulating a subjectivity—a body of feelings, sensations, and activity ("stretching, and / breaking . . . / splitting open") that shared authority with the more ego-driven or I-centered subject expressed in such conventionally narrative formulations as "I was pushing so hard at the end I was busting blood vessels in my face / so that I was pushing too hard and I had / you know / my eyes closed really tightly." The world Karen dis/composed, un/named was not divisible into light and dark, black and white, good and bad. It was a twilight world, a world of "waves" made imaginable but not exactly intelligible by the words she assigned to it.

Karen did not, as Scarry argues most people do, imagine her pain as injury or assault. For Scarry:

> There reappear again and again (regardless of whether the immediate context of the vocalization is medical or literary or legal) two and only two metaphors, and they are metaphors whose inner workings are very problematic. The first specifies an external agent of the pain, a weapon that is pictured as producing the pain; and the second specifies bodily damage that is pictured as accompanying the pain. Thus a person may say, "It feels as though a hammer is coming down on my spine" even where there is no hammer; or "It feels as if my arm is broken at each joint and the jagged ends are sticking through the skin" even where the bones of the arms are intact and the surface of the skin is unbroken. Physical pain is not identical with (and often exists without) either agency or damage, but these things are referential; consequently we often call on them to convey the experience of pain itself (SCARRY 1985:15).

Karen did not refer her pain to external means. Metaphorically, she wasn't done to; she did it. She did pain. Her images of opening and rending, moreover, suggested less wounding than release: an opening onto a space of feeling and knowing previously untouched by mind, body, or language. Here in this space pain consisted, she said, in "stretching, and breaking . . . / Splitting open and it [the baby] was coming out my anus." In these images Karen transgressed codes by which pain was bad (the enemy to be avoided and forgotten) and by which images of the body opening, splitting, and expelling—especially by identification with the excremental function of the anus—are taboo.[14] This was a violent representation, a representation of the body ripping and tearing that itself simultaneously tore at what Kristeva has called "weavings of abstractions" and, for all intents and purposes, fulfilled Kristeva's charge to women writing: to "let a body venture at last out of its shelter, take a chance with meaning under a veil of words." She wrote her-self, her pain and pleasure, in what Kristeva (in another context) calls "word flesh," the concrete flow of images and metaphors that constitute "an ordeal discourse, like love." "What is loving, for a woman," writes Kristeva, is "the same thing as writing" (Kristeva 1986b:162).

This was an ordeal. It was by no means easy. It was as difficult as loving/writing made more difficult, and more pleasurable, by direct contact with an other, by the performative immediacy of touching, looking, grazing another's arm in the awkward process of "passing off" the baby while swiping spills and crumbs from the counter that, like most borders, divided/joined Karen and me. Karen braced her pain with the colloquial image of "seeing these stars" and the somewhat more elevated appeal to riding "waves." But even in weaving these hybrid forms into her body-text she continued to challenge the conventionally unitary representation of the body as an object or of the birthing woman as the passive victim of overwhelming aggressive pain. She continued to rip at the fabric of pain as the just penance for female sexuality / sensuality and, in "word flesh," at once to open and begin to rewrite the discourses by which birth pain is and will be understood.

Practicing pain in this way, Karen set herself up for two other kinds of practice, material and critical: she practiced or rehearsed the subject/self she would perform in her next birth and she, with new license, challenged the class relations and class *pain* that overtook her hospital stay.

It just so happened that Alan had wandered into the kitchen while we were talking. He proceeded to fix a sandwich, imagining us in a conversation to which he had previously—in other forms, at other times—been privy. But as Karen reached what she called the "worst part" of the story, the part about a nurse's crude ministrations after the birth, she nervously indicated embarrassment at his presence. "This is hard for me to say . . ." she said, glancing at Alan. He left—and she felt her sense of modesty sufficiently restored to recount how much more violated it had once been:

> **KAREN:** Well, she gave me these pads and these net underwear things and
> then she said (*sharp tone*), "Do this, this, this and this."
> And . . . and, and I tried to do it. And she said (*angrily*), "I didn't say put that in the trash can, I didn't say put that in here."

DELLA: You're kidding.

KAREN: I said (*voice high and fast*), *You didn't say where to put it, I,
           I, I've never done this before you know* and I started to
           get really

           upset, you know just like sad and feeling really stupid. It
           was *awful*, it was awful, I couldn't control the stuff
           coming out of me.

           "Stand on the toilet!" you know (*voice high and fast*), *I
           thought you wanted me to do this, I'm sorry* . . . and
           then, after a while, it was just like I'm sorry, I'm sorry.

DELLA: Oh, God.

KAREN: Kept doing everything wrong.

           It was just awful. Yeah.

           "Put that in here!"

           (*laughs*)

           She *introduced* herself you know and said, "Do this,
           this and this."

           And then I (*laughing*) didn't do it right. It was awful.
           It was awful.

           I was afraid to ask her any

           questions. I didn't know *what* she was *talking* about.

           I didn't know what, what the *goal* was, what was I
           trying to do.

           You know and I would say, "Am I supposed to change
           this every you know so often, am I supposed to, uh
           what am I . . . " and she would, she would just

           you know, answer me real shortly

           like I was supposed to know, like I knew and I was just
           giving her a hard time.

DELLA (*laughs*):

           She *told* you!

KAREN: Yeah, she told me.

           I didn't . . .

           Like I

           was supposed to get it and I didn't, it was awful.

           You know it was just me and her

           in the bathroom.

           I was just . . . it was bad (*baby coos over the conversation*).
           And I'm so modest anyway . . . I had just had a baby

> and I just didn't . . .
> it was awful.

DELLA: And she was just kind of
manhandling you?

KAREN (*angrily*):
"Put that in the toilet!" You know she wouldn't help me.
It was, it was so *gross* she couldn't stand it or something,

DELLA: Oh, God!

KAREN: or, or I was supposed to know what I was doing and I
was stupid or . . .
and I just thought I was *stupid*. I really did think I . . .
and I wasn't, now that I think
about it.

DELLA: Of *course* not.
Why would you know any of this?

KAREN: I don't know (*high voice, laughing*), *I don't know*!
I didn't get *angry* I just felt sad and stupid, you know, I
didn't get angry.
Next time I'm just getting angry (*both laugh*)! I'll say
Get outta here!
"Get out of my room right now!" You know (*laughing*),
push her out!

DELLA: Good! Ooo, I want to see this (*laughs*)!

KAREN: I would, but I, I, I didn't.
I just felt stupid.
I wanted to cry.

Here, if anywhere in Karen's story, was the account of pain as injury—of physical control, humiliation, and punishment used to discipline Karen's subjectivity, to re/produce her in the image of the nurse's expectations.[15] The nurse literally charged the borders of Karen's body. She followed Karen into the bathroom, where she pushed her, with aggressive disregard for modesty or privacy, into apologetic submission. "It was awful," Karen said, "I couldn't control the stuff coming out of me. / "Stand on the toilet!" *I thought you wanted me to do this*, I'm sorry / and then, after a while, I was just like I'm sorry, I'm sorry." The nurse used Karen's body against her. She made Karen "feel really stupid" for its excesses and vulnerability, effectively putting what Karen felt so sharply as a lack of control on display before her condemning eyes. In fact, she made Karen feel so stupid that Karen assumed she was / is stupid. As Karen said, "She was mean and I'm stupid." The nurse *made* her stupid. She was mean, Karen felt stupid, Karen was stupid. I was staggered by the speed with which the nurse's behavior, operating as it did on and through the manipulation of Karen's body, became Karen's faltering subjectivity and sense of identity.

But if the nurse used her authority to discipline Karen into a particular subject-identity, then the interview proved a counterdiscipline that drew the opportunity for embodied reflexivity into a process of alternative identity formation. "I just thought I was *stupid*," Karen said, "I really did . . . and I wasn't . . now that I think / about it." Thinking about it now, in the context of the interview, Karen not only disidentified with the self she had become under the nurse's control but practiced another self/subject, another way of feeling and being. She turned everything the nurse made her feel was "gross" about her self/body into what she later called "rabid" assertiveness. She claimed the rights of excess, rehearsing now, in word and body, what she would do "next time":[16] "Next time I'm just getting angry (*both laugh*)! I'll say / Get outta here! / 'Get out of my room right now!' You know (*laughing*) *push* her out!" Karen vamped on the subjectivity she would practice some three, four months from now, in her next birth, the prospect of which gave her a material stake in the account of this one. "I'd say," she said, " 'I'm sorry you're having a bad day, but if you can't laugh and smile get out of here. / If you can't be even polite, then leave. Get out' (*laughs*). / I'll call security or I'll say 'you're . . .' I'll say . . . no, I don't know *what* I'd say, but I'm sure if I just said 'get out,' she'd *get out*."

I had no doubt that she would—and suddenly felt chilled, chided by the possibility of hearing this voice myself, of warranting—by the fact of occupying the position of both personal and economic power in our relationship that I did—this censure, this *push*. Why did the nurse—and the doctor after her, who insisted he didn't need a badge to take her baby away to the nursery, who seemed to feel no obligation either to identify himself to her or to respond to her arguments to the contrary—treat her like that? Where did they get the authority of their presumptions?

By way of an answer Karen imagined herself refracted through the nurse's gaze:

> I was young and I had these blood—blood—blood
> vessels busted
> —busted all over my face . . . I was Medicaid. I don't
> know if they

saw that on my chart but . . . Medicaid, young, ugly
you know, busted up face,
it was my first child, didn't know anything about
   newborns
except for what I learned in class, what I read—
I mean, I had *never* taken care of one—
so, I think that's why.

Seeing herself as she imagined the doctor and nurse must have seen her, reading what, through their eyes, became the text of her own body, Karen saw all the markings of "white trash." She was young—she might have been seventeen, eighteen, one more teenage mother, the poor, stupid white girl whose broken blood vessels (the effect of pushing so hard during delivery that the veins in and around her eyes popped, leaving her face bruised and swollen) made her not only physically but socially ugly, dirty, gross. Accordingly, it was she—not they—who had now violated codes of femininity, whose bruises rose like stigmata on her face, making visible (following Victorian and Puritan mandates for madonnalike births) the contaminant, wanton self hidden inside her woman's body. The "truth" was "out." She must be disciplined. Read from the outside in, she was no longer the powerful woman who rode out crashing "waves" of pain to give birth but the "busted up" object of brutality, a victim, like the victim of domestic violence, whose bruises are so repulsive they invite judges and juries to wonder whether she didn't in fact deserve whatever she got, to distinguish unfavorably between her plight and the plight of a woman presumed to be because more visibly "pure" and to run from whatever responsibility or implication they might otherwise see in the mirror her face held up to them.

Linked to her Medicaid status, gender pain became class pain became race pain. Not knowing for sure exactly how or where Medicaid showed up on her chart, how it was graphed into her body/history, but "sure that it shows up somewhere at the hospital," Karen felt herself subject to reprisal for dependence on public funding.[17] With pride and some defensiveness, she first insisted, reiterating by negation demon narratives of welfare "queens" that permeated the press and politics at the time: "I'm not actually on welfare." Then, backing up to defend black women who, like her, received Medicaid support, she argued, "Black women get really / they get really discriminated against. It's awful." Karen went on to describe differences in breastfeeding instruction and patient care she'd witnessed, explaining, "It's not because it's a white nursing staff or a black nursing staff. It's just because / they're Medicaid and they're black. . . . It's like a stereotype." Karen challenged the stereotype and yet, implicitly, repeated another. Pivoting on Medicaid, Karen identified by class (in her case, the particular substratum of class defined by the use of Medicaid vs. welfare) across raced differences but disidentified with women on welfare generally, leaving them to the "disgusted look" one of the women with whom I spoke faced when she applied to Social Services for AFDC.[18]

Listening to Karen, I remembered one prenatal instructor's dismissal of the laboring women who arrived at the hospital emergency room without what she took to be sufficient prenatal education. In a half-whisper she invited us into smug satisfaction with our own lessons learned: *Seventy-five percent of the women we get down there don't know a thing—half the time, they don't even know they're pregnant.* Hushed as it was, this shared secret seemed meant to make us feel that we—all middle-class, mostly white men and women—were privileged by the very knowledge we were gaining in her course. It consolidated knowledge, class, and power in a phrase—and suggested that Karen's sense that the black women she knew had it worse than she did may have been most significant in marking her white, in clarifying her precarious position in a hierarchical system that is, as Karen observed, based in the stereotypical equation of black, poor, and ignorant. White and poor, Karen embodied a contradiction untenable within the hospital hierarchy—confusing a system that relied on the exclusive identification of black and poor to secure white middle-class privilege—and so came in, it seemed to me, for special reprisals, for the nurse's vexed orders, for the doctor's stubborn refusal to recognize that she knew what he knew: that his authority rested less in his body per se than in his missing badge. Karen had to be made to fit. She had to be *made* stupid, even as Margaret was *made* crazy. She was punished, I think, at least in part, for sliding on a scale that was supposed to be fixed.

Karen's pain was public pain. It was expressed against (flat in the face of) discursive bans on the birthing body; articulated in and through other stories exchanged in public settings as a matter of informal public record, felt, changed, and shaped in relation to the people who attended her birth, and conditioned by her position within class/knowledge formations that delimit desire and require "stupidity."

As such, it engaged the performative power of pain. Various scholars have shown how pain fuses "emotional/physical states with the ideological organization of the social structure" to shape identity.[19] Karen's performance, however, refuses an easy identification of the self with the institutions that regulate pain. It is disruptive and disjunctive. It forces a gap between social construction and self-making, suggesting, as Nadia Seremetakis argues, that "the personal communication of pain, synthesizing emotional force and body symbolism, can vividly dramatize the dissonance between self and society. This discontinuity can attain a collective dimension by exploiting the moral capacity of emotional inference to generate affective enclaves" or what she calls "communities of pain and healing."[20] In and as performance, Karen's story demarcates existing social structures and calls new, shifting sets of social relations into being/becoming. It claims the social idiom of pain for its own purposes, heralding a space in which speaking pain is not only a formidable technique for making alternative selves but an ethic of community formation, a moral/emotional language compelling the performance of counterselves and collectivities.[21]

* * * *

I often used Andrea's story as a horror story. I would invite listeners into the morbid pleasure of knowing that this was the "worst," that this story set such a clear and distant horizon for pain that anything else seemed/would seem mild. I'd set it up for its sheer narrative value. "Listen to *this* one," I'd say or imply, the horror never lets up: just when you think it's as bad as it gets, it gets worse. I'd then tell it in three quick punches, reducing the three-times trauma it held to something like a good joke.

Andrea had told me her story as a cautionary tale. It was meant to be passed on—but she didn't particularly want to tell it, to me or to anyone. She did because I asked and, secondarily, because she thought someone else, somewhere might benefit from hearing it. She wasn't one of those women who "needed" to tell it, she insisted. She didn't speak for herself but for me and for unnamed others, in the name of their possible pain. For Andrea, the story was a reluctant warning. It was her attempt to qualify the norms of expedience that seemed to lead more and more women and physicians to choose cesarean section and to which she felt she had succumbed.

Andrea was carrying twins. Both were breech. She'd been chronically nauseous for nine months (evoking the permeation of every body/space boundary by vomit, she said, "I had a bowl, I had a bowl, by the bed, / I had a bowl in the car, I had a bowl underneath my desk"). Still, she continued to work full-time as a lawyer in a large company, suffering not only nauseating office smells and chatty pep talks that, each in their own way, made her want to throw up, but the example of a colleague who sat through a seven-hour deposition, seven months pregnant, without eating, and lived to tell it—proudly. She came home to the care of her three-year-old daughter while her husband, David, a GI (gastrointestinal) fellow at a Chicago area hospital, met his "third night" (all night, every third night) call schedule.

Andrea knew that trying to deliver breech twins vaginally would be difficult and especially risky for the second baby. Out of fear and with good reason, she planned to deliver by cesarean section. But she also recognized that, somewhere in the back of her mind, she'd assumed a cesarean would be easier, that it would be a relief. Physically and emotionally depleted, she warmed to the idea that a cesarean would be less work. "I had wanted a C-section 'cause I was afraid for the second twin," she began, "but after what I went through / I would *never encourage* anyone."[22] What she went through—including loss of breath from the double pressure of the babies' heads on her diaphragm, a kink in the IV cord that cut off the anesthetic mid-surgery, a distended colon (a not uncommon side effect of anesthesia that nonetheless threatened to burst under negligence), bursting abdominal stitches, an Ob/Gyn who claimed her insurance company insisted on an early discharge, not to mention two premature infants in special care—all seemed to leave Andrea ravished, hollowed out by pain. She seemed numb now not because she felt too little but because she felt too much. From the outset overwhelmed by feeling, the birth drew Andrea back from feeling to a near-death state, to what David Morris has called a "zero degree where pain and sensation vanish together," leaving her now not without pain but without sufficient power to feel it and, in feeling it, to name it, and in naming it, to know it and, knowing it, to own it (Morris 1991:116).[23]

Andrea seemed lost to her accumulated pain even as she mourned the loss of a creative life. She had wanted to be a writer. She'd studied fiction and poetry writing before law school. But she never read and rarely wrote anymore, although the possibility of some day or late night finding enough time and energy to steal away to the computer hidden in a basement closet seemed to keep her desire alive. (Thinking back to Karen and her painting: did Andrea's desire for children in some way create this desire? could it be —even echoing Kristeva's sense that one does not give birth *in* pain but *to* pain—that one does not give birth *in* desire but *to* contradictory, excessive, equally painful and pleasurable *desires*?) We sat upstairs, in the small living room, each absentmindedly rocking one of the babies asleep in the car seats at our feet. Each baby woke in turn. Andrea fed one and then the other, and then both; in between she offered me seconds on pound cake and wondered what else she could get me while I swept crumbs from the pillows and felt the afternoon sun begin to burn through the deck windows. Everything was too bright and too quiet. I felt I couldn't quite hear properly. That the story Andrea told came wrapped in cotton, even packed in gauze, like the incision on her abdomen that had eventually opened, broken its stitches, and promised terrible infection.

I feel compelled now to quote Andrea's story at length, to give it the space for which it was intended but which her voice could never quite inhabit—and which my voice tended to diminish in horror story sound bites. Andrea's story came to me from some place far away. From a place of profound loss or perhaps of desire just temporarily locked away, like the computer in the basement closet. It was spectral in its precise evocation of a body literally cut off—by surgical trauma and negligence—from speech. Courteous, concerned, cautious (Andrea seemed caught between the fact and prospect of legal injuries: she charged her obstetrician with malpractice and yet protected herself against the libel charges that could follow), the story left me, ultimately, angry and frustrated—angry at the people and practices that effectively displaced Andrea in her own story and frustrated with Andrea for no cause of her own, for not having a cause, yes, I know, for not *being able* to speak up, for being the object of other's administrations, for being susceptible to being ignored, for representing desire blocked by countless others—her husband, her obstetrician, hospital administrators, insurance companies, the twins themselves, and even her body, as radically othered as it had been and seemed now. My frustration was deep and unfair, born, I'm sure of deep identification. Listening to Andrea's story, I could have been her, I was her, I am. After listening, I struggled, dumbfounded, for words, and found myself turning, uneasily, to the all-too-easy, domesticating form of the horror story. I'm struggling now to tell her story without overtelling it, without betraying it with my own anger, undercutting it, or speaking for her again, speaking over her voice, even as she was repeatedly spoken for/overwritten in the twins' birth.[24] I can only imagine being half-mute together, recognizing that pain lingers in this spoken silence, that here, in the intense detachment with which she performed her birth story, is the pain of the pain—not in the wounds that have now, fortunately, healed but in the split between Andrea's body and her voice and the words that trailed—relentlessly—in the breach:

I mean it was . . . from the beginning it was bad.
For one thing I got so big I had trouble breathing—
I *cannot breathe.*
Then they go to give me the epidural . . .
you lose your feeling from quite high up
from like your mid-chest point, and that complicated
my
feeling of I can't breathe. So I was in the operating
room and I'm
like "*I can't breathe*" and I had an oxygen mask on.
I had a very good anesthesiologist . . .
umm and you just *feel* like you can't breathe because the
twins are pressing on your diaphragm, two heads are
breech, and you're sort of paralyzed from the mid-
chest.
It was . . . it was *frightening!* I mean it was really
frightening!
I felt like
. . . and David was right there and he was watching the
monitor. He said,
The oxygen in your blood was fine . . .
"the oxygen in your . . . in your *blood* is fine!"

The first person who looked at me was the anesthesiology
resident. And I
swear she . . . she was like
(*very cheerful*): "Hi! How ya doing?" and she's like
(*mocking*) "Let's see, *where* should we put this
epidural?"

DELLA: Oh no! (*laughter*)
ANDREA: That's what I get for trying to deliver in a teaching
hospital . . . a resident practicing on me.
But then we did have a wonderful anesthesia
attending who came and actually *stayed.*
DELLA: Was that . . . was that standard that they would bring in
the attending?
ANDREA: I think they did it because of David. I really do.
DELLA: Oh.
ANDREA: That was really good. And I was saying "I, I just can't
breathe"

and they said "It's just the sensation."
Then, you actually . . . you cannot feel pain, but you
actually *feel* them pulling.

DELLA: So you . . . so for the C-section all you had was the
epidural?

ANDREA: But a real strong one.

DELLA: A real strong one.

ANDREA: Yeah, a *real* strong one. I mean . . . from *mid*-chest
I didn't feel any pain.
. . . but then you feel this *tugging*! I mean like somebody
is really *tugging*!
You can feel them.
They, they drape you so you can't see it,
but you can *feel* them.
The point that they're *pulling* apart the muscles and
trying to get the baby—

I mean it's really awful !

DELLA: And they literally . . . I guess that's literally what
they're doing.

ANDREA: What they're doing
yeah what they're doing.
Now *maybe* because I was so stretched out
and there was just no room there,
maybe it was . . .

DELLA: Did you have a sensation of being cut?

ANDREA: A lot of pressure.
You, you don't feel like someone is *cutting*
but you feel a lot of pressure.

Now, then the *line* into my spine got *kinked*
and then I *did* feel pain. I felt a sharp pain.
That was also frightening.
David told me this, that the line got kinked.
They, they put nitrous oxide on me (*Della gasps*) and
tried to straighten out the line.

DELLA: But that sounds just like crazy . . . I mean that sounds
like . . .

ANDREA: It was . . . it was . . . it was yeah—just *terrible* (*laughs*)

I just, I just definitely—I had taken C-section so *lightly,*
and I would never recommend it.
Really,
They got the babies out
and you could hear 'em cry, one after another.

At that point, they won't give you any sedative.
I was begging them for Valium
before they got the babies out.
They gave me something else,
after, after they were delivered, yeah.
So *then,*
you're in the recovery room for a while and then they
    take you to the regular *room* and . . .
when you get back to your room they (*sighs*)
they give you a morphine pump . . .

DELLA: You can just keep pumping it into your system.
ANDREA: Well, it will only . . . there's a limit
like it will not dispense more than a certain dose every
    hour, type thing.
But you you have . . .
it is a manual control.

But where *I* started getting into trouble is that they had
loaded up the *epidural* with morphine
so that I would have more prolonged pain relief
But morphine is,
being a narcotic,
one of its side effects is that it
(*slowly*) essentially paralyzes your colon.
So I had morphine in the epidural,
and then I had morphine . . .
I wasn't giving myself very *much* morphine,
because I wasn't feeling a lot of pain.
Then also just the physical act of opening up . . .
the *surgery* of a C-section: once you get air inside the
cavity that also can
contribute to the paralysis.

DELLA: Oh.

ANDREA: So I um
          had the C-section on Friday, and on Sunday
          I looked like I was nine months pregnant, my
              stomach was so distended.
          And, what was starting to happen was that our
              obstetrician *missed*
          an important complication.
          And she's a *seasoned* obstetrician.
          So she comes in to see me,
          and she, she prescribes,
          (right now I'm on nothing by mouth)
          she prescribes two *oral* uh laxatives and a heating pad
          and leaves.
          And, I mean, *luckily* I was a married to a fellow in GI,
          'cause David came and looked at me
          and said, "This is a *terrible* situation!"
          And I had a basically, a severe, um
          it's called an ileus,
          the beginnings of a severe *bowel* complication.
          So *he* was put in the *bad* position of having to . . .
          interfere in the case!
          So he talked to the OB resident and said "Look, I'm a
              GI fellow; she has an ileus; I think you should have
              her have an X-ray!"
          And this . . . the the . . . the obstetrician missed
              completely.
          And then finally the OB *resident agreed* that I should
              have an X-ray and
          agreed that the the obstetrician's advice to simply take an
              oral laxative just
          wasn't gonna go anywhere because my *bowel* was
              paralyzed.
          She recommended
          after talking to David
          that . . . the first thing you had to do is keep me on
              no liquids. *But*
          the other thing is he had told me is "*You must, you must*
              stop the narcotics."
          This was the second postoperative day . . .
DELLA: This was the resident? or David?

ANDREA: David!
that said you must stop the narcotics. And the resident
said "Nah! she
can take the narcotics."
And David said, "If *I* were called on a GI consult, I
would tell you you've
gotta stop it.
You're gonna *get* into *terrible* trouble."
So it was another thing, the one OB resident was
saying, ya know, it's OK, and *he* was saying you gotta
stop it .

DELLA: But this really is something within the GI specialty!

ANDREA: *That's* what he knows about
and I stopped it.
So I stopped taking the morphine on Sunday and I was
in excruciating pain.
Because that was the second day after the C-section.
But I figured he knew what he was doing. And what
happened was that
I had this terrible distension of the bowel and if it
had gotten *worse*, there
were a number of really gruesome things that they
would have
tried.
But I could have ended up losing
. . . being wheeled into surgery to have a portion of my
colon removed.
I mean, the worst-case scenario is that I could have
ended up with an
ileustomy.

So I, I stopped the narcotics and I was just delirious
with pain on Sunday.
And he called a friend of his and they, they rigged up
a combination of
Phenergen and Tylenol
which really doesn't have much pain-relieving
properties,
but the Phenergen is a sedative and I got through
Sunday night

and by Monday
I could endure being without the narcotics.
And *STILL* the obstetricians were saying if you're really in pain you can
take narcotics.
But I didn't
and I listened to him.

DELLA: Was that just defensive?

ANDREA: I think so.
I think they were—
and they *were*—being stupid!
I mean this was, this was
the makings of a good *malpractice* case.
And I'm not gonna *sue* them because I don't have any permanent damage.
Knock on wood.
But it was *classic,* because even when the OB resident had heard that the obstetrician had prescribed an oral laxative she
(*quietly and incredulously*) she couldn't *believe* it! I mean that's like
incompetence! I mean an *oral* laxative rather than . . .
there's no way that those laxatives were going to get anywhere.

DELLA: Did you end up talking with your OB about this?

ANDREA: Yeah,
well
well, what happened was that
they kept me off [food]:
nothing by mouth which was *very* difficult
'cause I was trying to nurse both babies. So I'm drinking nothing
and I was just so thirsty I could *scream.* Ya know, and finally
I *begged* them to put me on a clear liquid diet.
And again then David thought I should be X-rayed at certain points, and they
(*sarcastic*) the OB didn't think I needed to be X-rayed
and he was put in the uncomfortable *position* of having to be very *assertive.* I mean it was something that he

knew about. But to have to argue with these other
physicians about how your wife is being treated was
really difficult!
He had to really go out on a limb. And I,
I mean
he *saved* my colon by himself.
He's the only one who saw what was going on and
stopped it before it got worse!
I mean the OB would have just simply let me *slide* into
a *disastrous* complication.
I mean she didn't care,
(*deliberately*) she really didn't *care*!
So *then* on *Tuesday* I thought . . .
I was I still on clear liquids and I thought that,
Well, it's not getting any worse so that's good. It was
still very distended but it wasn't getting worse.

They take the staples of the incision out
and she comes in to look at the incision and she says, "It
looks good." Now David comes back that evening,
and looks at the incision and says, "I haven't seen a
surgical incision like this since I took obstetrics in
medical school in my third year. But this doesn't look
right."
So that night, he *called* the wife of a friend of his, who's
an obstetrician in the same group and said, "*Please*
could you do us a favor." And she didn't really know
us very well . . .
He said, "could you do us a favor, could you go look at
Andrea's incision." And she could've said no,
it was politically bad for her, this is something that
another obstetric
attending is supposed to be taking care of, but she
was . . .
she's a person that when I had met her the first time, I
really didn't (*disapprovingly*) care for her. I thought
she was sort of a loudmouth, aggressive . . . sort of a
bitch, ya know.
But, she went out on a *limb*!
She came by to my room and she looked at it,

she brought the chief resident with her.

She said, "You have a *problem* here, your incision has opened up,

and you've got a *big* problem here,

we're gonna have to . . . it's not gonna heal.

We have to determine how *deep* it is and whether

you have an infection going in there."

So what had happened is that the obstetrician had now missed a second

major complication.

DELLA: How could she be *missing* this?

ANDREA: I think she doesn't care, is what I think it is. I think she just didn't . . .

I mean she was an attending,

attending obstetrician. I think.

I mean,

I mean what had happened is, in about 10 percent of cases

—the stitches *don't hold.*

DELLA: Just because it was so big?

ANDREA: It could've been . . . and I had no muscle tone.

It *does* happen in obese women and it happens in women with multiple pregnancies.

It happens in some other women too, but not typically; it's only when there's a

complicating factor.

Probably because I had twins, I had no muscle tone, the stitches simply

opened up.

So what I had was the *incision*, the *hole*, from the baby.

DELLA: When your OB came in and looked at your incision there was an open incision there

and she didn't see it?

ANDREA: She didn't see what was wrong with . . .

DELLA: That there was raw tissue?

ANDREA: Yeah, that it was getting, beginning to get inflamed, and

what she *missed* was that the stitches had split and it was beginning to open up. So . . .

DELLA: That is *un*missable!
ANDREA: yeah, it is, it is unmissable
DELLA: . . . by just your everyday person.
ANDREA: It is! it is unmissable
            and it's
            it's medical malpractice.
            I mean it's *gross* incompetence.
            It's somebody who doesn't *care* about the patient,
            who just simply looked without looking.
            Ya know, just to,
            to have it show that she had done her rounds.

            And what they had to do,
            I mean it was basically a gaping hole the size of a . . .
            silver dollar and
            about like
            like, like an inch and a half *deep*.
            They had to determine *how* deep it was . . .
            down to the muscle layer (*Della gasps and moans*).
            So here I've got a hole,
            and *now* they can't just stitch it up
            because fluid will collect in there
            and you'll get like a *massive* pelvic infection.
DELLA (*sighs heavily*):
            Oh!!
ANDREA: So they have to resort to a sort of barbaric way of
                making it heal and that is
            by *packing* it.
            Now, I couldn't take any narcotics for the *pain* of *this*.
DELLA: Oh God!
ANDREA: I was just really . . .
            They had to *probe* it several times
            and then they had to,
            they had to *pack it* with
            um saline gauze three times a day. I mean and it
            just hurt
            like crazy. I mean it's just someone packing a hole in
            your stomach.
DELLA: Oh! it sounds so miserable!

ANDREA: Yeah. *Again*, David spotted it and
                um this friend of his went out on a *limb* because it was
                    very . . .
                I mean, she could've easily said, "No, it's too politically
                    sensitive."
DELLA: Forget your body just . . .
ANDREA: Yeah, but I'm *really* grateful to her for . . .
DELLA: What would've happened if it had not been perceived?
ANDREA: What would have *happened* is it would eventually
                    become a *massive* infection. I mean it could be a life-
                    threatening infection. It was, it was just *not* going to
                    heal by itself. It would've accumulated serum and
                    blood that would've become infected
                and I would've been in the hospital on IV antibiotics
                for a month.
                So *then*
                Ok I've got *this* now, that has to be packed.
                On *Friday* morning, a *week* after my surgery,
                I'm only on what they call
                full liquids at this point. I have eaten no solid food.
                They have *not* determined how my bowel will tolerate
                    solid food. The
                obstetrician,
                my obstetrician, the attending obstetrician comes in and
                    tells me that she going to discharge me the next day,
                    because the *insurance* company
                called her and they think I'm staying in the hospital
                    too long.
DELLA: This is the same one that . . .
ANDREA: The same one.
                And this is again, gross negligence
                because you can't discharge someone from the *hospital*
                    with a paralyzed
                colon without determining whether they can *tolerate*
                    solid food!
DELLA: So has the distension gone down at this point?
ANDREA: Some but not . . .
                it hasn't clinically resolved.
                David was following the X-rays.

	I mean, then . . .
	If she would send me home, I would eat something
	and I would go into a GI emergency and I would have
	to . . .
	at least my babies were in the hospital with me . . .
	I'd have to go back to the emergency room
DELLA:	Oh God!
ANDREA:	And who was going to take care of these two premature
	infants? They were
	still one month premature.
	She just wanted to dump me out.
	So I repeated that conversation to David, and he
	called her,
	he paged her and said,
	"You know, *surely* Andrea was mistaken. She mentioned
	that you were
	going to be discharging her tomorrow because of the
	insurance company."
	And she said, "No, no the insurance company is not going
	to prolong—is not going to pay for this any longer.
	And he said "OK, thank you." And he immediately
	called the chair of the department and *complained.*
DELLA:	Did he give the whole story?
ANDREA:	The whole story.
	And that afternoon the chairman of the department
	came in and very
	graciously (obviously he can't admit anything) he said,
	"We feel that you
	need to have a different physician."
DELLA:	*Good.*
ANDREA:	She was gonna dump me out!
DELLA:	That's unbelievable!!!
ANDREA:	Yeah! She just wanted to get me out
	she wanted to *get me* out from under her care,
	have me readmitted, ya know,
	on the GI floor
	with *two* premature infants.
	I mean just, I don't know . . .
DELLA:	But *admitted* under emergency care conditions.

                And the likelihood of that is tremendous.

ANDREA: It was tremendous!

                I don't know, I think maybe she started to *resent* David's
                    involvement?

                I think she's a lazy person who doesn't care.
                She was just tactless! She had said . . .
                I had *seen* her,
                she was one of five OB's . . .
                I had seen her several times,
                and she made a statement during that week I was in the
                    hospital like, uh
                "Oh well you know, I don't remember seeing you." She
                said that to me. I
                mean if you don't remember a patient, fine! you don't
                    remember a patient,
                but you don't tell them "I don't remember ever seeing
                you," and I had seen
                her several times.
                So . . . it was clear to me that she just didn't, did not
                    care at all.

DELLA: She was just checked out, I mean completely.

ANDREA: Yeah, and I was *very lucky*
                to have a husband who is a physician
                and that this other obstetrician went out on a limb
                    for me.
                I know that the chairman of the department also did
                    talk to her about the
                failure of the incision to heal.

                So,
                then they sent me home
                with a *wound* that had to be packed three times a day
                    for four to six weeks.

DELLA: Did David come home to do it?

ANDREA: What it was was that he,
                he would pack it
                at six in the morning, and then he would pack it
                    at like . . .

he tried to come home a little bit earlier.
He'd pack it at *five* at night and then pack it at midnight again.

DELLA: Oh!

ANDREA: I could've had a home health nurse come in, but he was
doing a good job
and knew what he was doing.
And having it packed at three in the afternoon
versus six
I didn't think made a difference.

DELLA: What *did* this do for your *mobility?*

ANDREA: Ohh! Alot of pain and ya know
I couldn't shower at all.

DELLA: Did you actually move with this?

ANDREA: I could walk around with it but um it was, it was *sore.*
I mean you have this ball of gauze stuck in your belly.
They [the babies] were so small that I could lift
them up,
but I couldn't bend over to load the dishwasher or any
thing. I just didn't
do anything at all but nurse them.
I mean you're just so *tired* as it is. I had all this stuff.
I mean
these are complications of a C-section,
I was unfortunate enough to get both of them.
They're not that common, but they *do* occur. And ya
know—
I always thought having a C-section would be something *easy,* but it's
not:
it's *major* surgery.
The recovery is hard and to the extent that people can
avoid them, I mean
three days in labor is no fun.
I know that you had a lot of pain with your delivery,
but getting around a C-section
if anyone can, it's really
the recovery is
so much prolonged over a vaginal delivery. You know?

DELLA: It sounds like,

like there was just so much emotional pain involved.
As a result of your care . . .
or lack of care.

ANDREA: I don't know what people do that don't have somebody
with a medical
background
watching them. Someone
that could pick these things up.

DELLA: It really does sound like David did a good job.

ANDREA: He did. . . .
Yeah. He really *saved* me.
He really did. I was lucky.
I was really lucky with having him.

Andrea is the absent figure in her own story. Flattened by pain, weighed down by a sense of her body as an object on which other people do or don't act, suffering the multiple injuries of neglect, being taught by neglect that she doesn't have enough presence in her own right even to be seen, even for her physician to notice her bloated gut or the infection gathering around the gaping hole in her abdomen, Andrea writes herself absent. She tells this story as if watching herself—intensely—from a great distance. As if, on the one hand, burned out by feeling too much and, on the other hand, deserted by feeling, numb even to her desire to breath, to speak. The last we hear from her directly is the muffled cry she issues from behind the oxygen mask covering her mouth and nose: "I can't breathe!" By this token her story is one of losing her voice to the devastations of her body. To the extent that she does speak in the scenes she recounts, she does so only by implication and as a cue for someone else to take action: "So I repeated that conversation to David . . . " she says of her response to the doctor's discharge orders, and, for the third time, David goes on to do for her what she cannot do herself.

Her pain remains oblique. For the most part she names her self and body through and for others. She sees herself as the object of her physician's and David's interventions and she presents herself as an object lesson for women who have not yet started down the "path" of medical interventions turned complications. In effect, even in speaking, Andrea seemed to be spoken for. Talked over and owned out. Even at the height of her critique she seemed absent, lingering behind David, hospital administrators, and her own torn and exhausted body in their competing efforts to be heard. In this sense the pain that radiated most forcefully from her story performance was the pain of absence, the pain of feeling her voice overtaken by her body and her body overtaken—for good and for ill—by medical practice.

Andrea's birth story became, in effect, not an illness narrative per se (a story usually structured either by the poles of trauma/recovery or the flat-line of chronic distress) but a surgery story, a story in which the distinctions between birth and illness collapsed in an account of what it means or can mean to cut open the human body.[25] This was a story about excision. Even Andrea's twin babies disappear under what seems the narrative pressure to observe her physician's crude incompetence and lack of care and to witness, in turn, her husband's careful mastery. They appear primarily as yet another complication ("she wanted to *get me* out from under her care, / have me readmitted, ya know, / on the GI floor / with *two* premature infants") that was nonetheless "small" enough to be barely manageable, small enough not to divert the narrative from its more pressing concerns. Reflecting on her return home, she refers to her babies as a lesser effort than loading the dishwasher ("They were so small that I could lift them up, / but I couldn't bend over to load the dishwasher or anything") that nonetheless consumed all of her remaining energy: "I just didn't / do anything at all but nurse them."

At the center of her story is the physician who "just simply looked without looking," who not only didn't remember *seeing* Andrea during one of several prenatal exams but, worse, "*said* that to me." She performed *not seeing, not remembering* on Andrea's body, diminishing her to nothing—a figment, a scrap—by what Eve Sedgwick calls one of the most expert forms of power: inattention (Sedgwick 1990).

The villains in Karen and Andrea's stories are women. Karen's nurses saw too much: they saw Karen as stupid and ugly and treated her accordingly, crudely manipulating the intimacies of birth and care. Andrea's physician saw nothing at all, not even the belly swollen with infection (and error) laid flat before her. Both Andrea and Karen raged against the women responsible for their care. To the extent that Andrea was grateful for the second Ob/Gyn's willingness to intervene, she was surprised: "She's a person that when I had met her the first time, I really didn't (*disapprovingly*) *care* for her. I thought she was sort of a / loudmouth, aggressive . . . sort of a bitch, ya know. / But, she went out on a *limb*! / She came by to my room and she looked at it." In other stories, it seems, the (female) nurses were nasty or nice; there was little in between. I don't know exactly what's going on here—whether the physical closeness and exposure in birth set especially high standards for care, whether professional jealousies and hierarchies (pitting nurses against physicians, obstetricians against physicians in male-dominated fields) get acted out on patients, whether women expect more and less from other women, depending on internalized misogynies or "natural"/naturalized affinities, whether the fantasy-memory of communal midwifery haunts the birthing room (like a romance of unrequited desire), whether women project their own sense of vulnerability and insufficiency onto their caregivers, whether, in the tradition of the Greek *doula,* new mothers want to be mothered and will find good mothers, evil stepmothers, and indifferent sisters wherever their narrative perspectives allow.[26]

I do know that, even in speaking against women, both Andrea and Karen spoke for women—and that both were lucky. Karen had the easiest birth anyone could imagine, especially by comparison to the pain she *had* imagined. David's expertise and assertiveness indisputably "saved" Andrea from more surgery, long-term damage, and even death. But what does it mean for Andrea to imagine David her savior, her white knight who rescues her from all kinds of female error? What does it mean for her to tell his story as her own, what is not in fact the "whole story" (as she claims he tells the department chair) but the story of how he *named* her body and, in naming it (representing it to other doctors and administrators), cured it, drew it back from the vertigo of pain and disease?

Andrea reiterates conventional narratives of heterosexuality. Her story is a story of David's professional dilemma and expertise. She is deeply invested in the risks he took for her, in the extent to which both he and his colleague went "out on a limb" for her, and in the professional norms they did not so much violate as restore in the process. Not only does David save her from the rampages of her body (in effect, saving her from her embodied self) but he provides the knowledge she needs to hold her fear at bay. In fact, his knowledge displaces her feelings. In telling her story she began to describe how afraid she was on the operating table, how paralyzed and on the very edge of death she felt, and then deferred to David's assurances that she was fine. She started to say, "I felt like . . . " started to exert the force of emotional/moral inference, moving from the declaration of feeling to its meaning for her and for me, listening to her, and then immediately fell, as if off the edge of narrative paralysis, into an account of what David said and did. She said, "I felt like," skipped to "and David was right there and he was watching the monitor," and then deferred to his ability to *see* what she couldn't *feel.* She buried her voice in his reassurances—"He said, 'The oxygen in your blood was fine . . . the oxygen in your . . . in your *blood* is fine!'"—and for a moment after the minor hilarity of the perky new anesthesiology resident was replaced by an attending physician, "he" became "we": "But then we did have a wonderful anesthesia attendant who came and actually *stayed*."

Andrea repeatedly ran up against her gratitude to David. Time and again, just as her strength began to rise, just as her narrating self threatened to break the limits imposed on the self she narrated, she withdrew into gestures of appreciation. "I think they did it because of David. I really do," she said. And later: "I mean / he *saved* my colon by himself. / He's the only one who saw what was going on and / *stopped* it before it got worse!" And again: "Again, David spotted it . . . He really *saved* me. / He really did. I was lucky. / I was really lucky with having him." She concluded, "I mean, David has been a saint."

The image of David as a saint flowed into another metaphorical current, that of the path. Andrea pictured both her own anxiety and her concern for women who might approach a C-section lightly as a path down which she felt herself ineluctably drawn. Telling her story, she stood at the head of that path, warning other women to beware:

> The frightening thing about the hospital is that
> once you start to have problems, you really don't realize
>   how quickly stuff can just
> *fall apart*. You know, that's the thing: you just
>   don't realize,
> You just don't realize how quickly something like
> a mildly distended colon can become a *catastrophe*
> and you end up wearing a bag for the rest of your life.
>   That can happen very fast
> and you just don't appreciate the magnitude . . .
> or a simple infection can be something that threatens to
>   kill you. That's the
> frightening thing.
> That things can escalate.

DELLA:	So, during this, you're facing these disastrous consequences. I mean just . . .
ANDREA:	They're not that *likely*, it's just that they can happen.
DELLA:	But it did sound so *close*.
ANDREA:	You know, you . . .
	it's like a progression of things that go wrong. You just don't . . .
	it was more likely than not I was . . .

everything was going to resolve.
Once you start going down that path,
complications sort of spring up in your face and um
unless you've got *really* good people keeping an eye on
    it, it just gets out of control. I mean if if if David
had not spotted the bowel thing, it wouldn't have been
    discovered until I
had perforated my colon or something . . .
or was just in such severe pain that it had progressed
    from a
a *severe* ileus to a *disastrous* one.

For Andrea the path is the course not so much of chaos as of dependency. It is the way of surgical trauma requiring surgical control, the way of the "cure" reproducing itself in such need that Andrea became dependent on a kind and degree of medical "care" that had already proven itself unpredictable, out of control. Andrea was, in effect, demolished by an ironic run on medical authority. By authority undoing itself in the excesses of its own application, proving itself more excessive, more wanton, than the excessive female body on which its gaze is otherwise trained.[27]

The path also describes her narrative passage over and past her/a ghost body. With the exception of a few, pointed references to what must have been excruciating pain—the twisted anesthetic cord, the feeling of the doctors "tugging" at her open uterus—Andrea does not address the erosions, transformations of her own body. As if paying dues, she turns her story with her body over to David. Her subject/self slips away in vague generalizations and passive constructions:

it's like a progression of things that go wrong. You just don't . . .
it was more likely than not I was . . .
everything was going to resolve.

She does not or cannot finish either the assertion "You just don't . . ." or the assessment "it was more likely than not I was . . . " She stops just short of conclusions, resorting to the passive happy ending: "everything was going to resolve." She pastes over the probability that she was going to be fine and the shadow possibility that she might not be, even to the point of abandoning her "I" self, quietly, assuredly slipping it into the protective arms of "everything." "I was . . .": what was it that she could not/would not say? The end of her own story seems out of her hands. It is clear, however, in the repeated insistence on a path, a course, a progression that there will be an end, that the story—despite or beyond, in excess of herself—will come to closure. Suggesting a melancholy confidence in knowing at least this (or, above all, this), she seems willing to wait on fate: "everything was going to resolve."

Andrea seemed lost between the implications of her two main metaphors: between what seemed the inevitable course of medical complications she suffered and the almost overwhelming gratitude she felt toward David for recovering her from "that path." Despite the vehemence with which she criticized her physician, her own voice ("I mean and it just hurt / like crazy. I mean it's just someone packing a hole in your stomach") is subordinated to a twin sense of doom and good fortune, a sense of being powerless to overcome a tragic course of worsening complications without the almost surreal good luck she had in being married to someone allied with the hospital administration, who happened to be specializing in gastrointestinal disorders. More than the poles around which the story develops, the images of the path and of the husband/father/doctor as a saint seemed the lock and key on Andrea's story, the structural elements that bound her and, in the act of telling her story, continued to bind her to a pattern of gratitude and despair.

What are the implications of these metaphors for Andrea and perhaps for her listeners? In their important book, *Metaphors We Live By*, George Lakoff and Mark Johnson argue that metaphors not only pervade everyday language use but guide our everyday lives and action. Rather than merely dressing up "ordinary" language, metaphors give feeling, order, and direction to our lives. Buried in everday and conventional use, they code and shape how we think and act in the world. Metaphors speak from and to the body. They are, for Lakoff and Johnson, concrete ways of thinking. Insofar as they align an abstract concept with a familiar and sensuous one (e.g., time is money—"You need to *budget* your time"—or love is a difficult journey —"our marriage is *on the rocks*"—or argument is war—"He *shot down* all of my arguments," "His criticisms were *right on target*"), they merge the world of ideas with the world of feeling and action and translate *knowing* into *doing* (Lakoff and Johnson 1980:4).[28] In this way they take on what James Fernandez calls a performative aspect: they "pass over into performance"; "they provide images in relation to which the organization of behavior can take place" (Fernandez 1986:20, 7).

Andrea's metaphors bear ways of continuing to think and to act. In constructing her past as a path from which she was fortuitously delivered, she reproduces the structures of dependency, passivity, and gendered sub-ordination that defined her birth experience. She warns other women away. She expresses flat-out, burning anger in one turn and, in the next, casual disregard for medical directives ("having it [her incision] packed at three in the afternoon versus six / I didn't think made a difference"). And yet she condenses her absence and incapacity into metaphors that, as metaphors, transfer one field of experience into another, paving the very course she wants to challenge. Speaking or speaking out does not in itself guarantee freedom or redemption. As Carol Tavris says, "We can be imprisoned by stories; or we can be liberated by them" (Tavris 1992:309). Telling her story, Andrea drew the twists and turns of her particular "path" into narrative form. She told a story she did not want to tell but could not, once asked, *not* tell. A story stuck now, it seemed, in the groove of its own complications. Retelling, repeating it, Andrea seemed to give herself over to it—impassively, relentlessly—as if her own subjection were the toll paid for warning other women off the same course.

But the last moments of our conversation suggested the possibility of an alternative authority, a performative practice of pain founded in repe-tition with a *difference*. Suddenly, for a moment, Andrea seemed to throw off the mantle of stoic suffering she seemed destined to wear and to name in dialogue not so much her physical pain as the pain of deference and obligation she'd borne. In these last moments she was who she imagined. She narrated herself into being-as-becoming the person who once said what she would soon say: "Fine! *Do* it!!" she finally burned, enacting above all pleasure in the possibility of saying it again, her desire to say it again, calling her body to her words now in a performance of something like "word flesh" and yet hesitating at a point just past indebtedness. Andrea tempered her complaints with praise for David and struggled both in our conversation and in the scene she described to be "fair." And yet, for the first time, at the close of our conversation, she seemed to "take a chance with meaning under a veil of words." She seemed to let her body "venture at last out of its shelter" and in no uncertain terms to speak its hard truths. She betrayed her own image of David as a saint by describing a scene in which he proved himself utterly human by showing neither saintly patience nor superhuman generosity. Andrea simultaneously declared a critical and decisively *im*patient (bad patient?) "I," freeing them both from foreclosure within the roles of redeemer and redeemed, man and wife/mother. It was Andrea who now merited the special praise she tend-ed to reserve for others: she was "out on a limb," taking the risk, defying the gender/medical norms that claimed her with all the force of gravity, claiming her body now, if only in rights to exhaustion, exasperation, and blame:

ANDREA: It's a real up and down thing. I mean,
my moods are really
explosive and then quiet and then explosive. I mean,
sometimes I'll just get
. . . I'll just get so *fed up* from the *whole*
pregnancy bit.
And the disruption too.
I mean, David has been a saint. But the one thing he
just hasn't
experienced is the
total . . .
you just drop out of a normal life for a *year*! And
you begin to lose patience with that.
And I mean, you know, and like last night, I made him
get up.
I mean, it was one-thirty,
I had been up *till* twelve-thirty and Matthew started
crying at one-thirty
and I *couldn't* get out of bed. I mean I just let him *cry*.
And David finally said,
"I'm gonna get up and give him a bottle." And I said,
"Fine! *Do* it!!"
I mean, I just couldn't get up!
DELLA: Like physically? Just cannot . . .
ANDREA: Yeah, I just cannot get up.
I would imagine it's probably a depressive element too.
And like I just—I
had been with them, and they were crying since twelve-
thirty and you
know, they had drifted off for maybe forty-five minutes,
and then they were crying again. And um, you know, so,
from one thirty to two,
he's fussin' with them.
He'd been on *call*,
Tuesday night

and it really wasn't fair for me to do that.

DELLA: Still . . . He's used to being on call! (*laughs*)

ANDREA: He had been on the phone
          and had to go in,
          I mean it wasn't *fair* for me to do that *at all*.
          But, I just, I just couldn't get up, you know?

DELLA: It sounds like—I mean, there just comes a point where
          you're just not supposed to hold yourself to standards
          of fairness and rationality.

ANDREA: Yeah, you're just like saying "*Too bad!*"

* * * *

If I have learned anything about pain from listening to women tell birth stories, it is that pain is ordinary. Not in the sense of universal or so elemental as to collapse different kinds, interpretations, experiences of pain into one ultimate experience and so either to enable its easy dismissal (as in: it's nothing new, nothing special, it hurts but it hurts everyone) or to promote a unitary identification of "woman" with pain that replicates the masculine/feminine, culture/nature split that has so often been used against particular women. Nor in the utterly banal sense of ordinary as common or vulgar, a sense that seems to animate efforts to elicit men's empathy by comparing giving birth to shitting a basketball or, with a somewhat more organic though equally round and orange twist, a pumpkin. Or suggesting, as my prenatal instructor did, that the pain of giving birth is like what you might feel were you to pull your lower lip up over your head. Or answering a man's inquiry about what it was like by picturing, as one woman did, "this six-inch-wide belt that has all these little nails in it just wrapped around your abdomen and just getting tight, just pulled tighter and tighter and tighter and tighter."[29] And certainly not in the sense of normal as a standard by which variation is found deficient. Rather, I think of pain now as ordinary in Mary Russo's sense of feminism as an "ordinary" practice, as "heterogeneous, strange, polychromatic, ragged, conflictual, incomplete, in motion, and at risk" (Russo 1994:vi).

Birth stories practice pain *differently*. They mark it variable, shifting, doubled up and over again. They not only recount bodily risk but risk uncertainty and ambivalence in the act of representing pain. They unfix pain, loosing it from moorings in discourses of control and efficiency, suggesting that it may but does not necessarily mean either horror or, in a narrowly physiological sense, nothing at all. Rather than leveling women in identification with birth as a "space of abjection and risk," as a space of horror or meaninglessness or both, in which they are, in effect, horrible women, birth stories recall abjection and risk to a politics of the grotesque, to the power of "possibility and error" embodied if not in the birth itself then in the act of telling it (Russo 1994:29).

In performance pain is itself at risk: it is in danger of exploding into a thousand fragments and flashes of what it means and might mean across a broad spectrum of public/private concerns. It is at risk of entering time, of being torn from memory (either forgotten there or tied to the past as such) in the act of remembering. In the time of remembering it is "ragged, incomplete, in motion." It is a figure of trespass, unpredictably turning away from the twin mythos of medicine and gender for the plainer pleasures of telling. In ordinary time, in the im/mediacy of telling pain, pain "unfolds time as difference and as radical heterogeneity" (Feldman 1991:2). Performed beyond the boundaries of anatomical discourse and its capacity to annihilate pain as meaning by dissecting and isolating it to segmented body parts or reflexes (in effect, by the rule of "divide and conquer"), pain exceeds medical/masculine distinctions in a surplus confabulation that is dense with the possibility of renewing body-meaning in diverse modes of practicing—rehearsing, reviewing, doing—pain. Remembered, remembering, it is not singular or even double but "heterogeneous, strange, polychromatic."

It is everyday:

> . . . I'm going, Oh, they're cramps (*laughter*)
> Oh (*laughter*), oh, oh, now I know what a contraction
>   is, it's
> a cramp. OK; yeah, a big cramp!
>
> —RACHEL[30]

> It was a blue pain.
> I see, I see pains in colors—and *real* intense pain
> it's like the top of a flame (*laughs*).
> You know the blue pain is always the most intense . . .
>
> —DENISE[31]

It is perverse:

> I felt like somebody was literally
> pulling my pelvic bone off.
>
> —YVONNE[32]

... part of me just felt like this isn't fair. This just hurts
too much.

—JANET[33]

It is diffuse:

the epidural felt really weird
because they put me on my side
and
I couldn't be on my back 'cause I hadn't slept on my
    back in months so
I couldn't get comfortable on my back.

I just felt, I sort of felt out of control ...
Every so often I was supposed to shift from one to the
other ... so, so my circulation would be OK? and
    so people,
Mark and the nurse, had to
shift me?
'cause I couldn't.
I couldn't move myself.
I think my arms weren't strong enough or something?
'Cause the only
things I had were my arms.
I couldn't roll myself over ... 'Cause I was *numb* from
my belly
button down.

And it felt really strange and my grandmother's in a
wheelchair now and
I kept on thinking about her and now I understood
how *depressed* she was 'cause all the time people had
to dress her and all
this stuff and it was just a really weird feeling ...

—ELYSE[34]

It is raced, erased:

This one nurse
was just the most *aaggravating*—
person. She, she just wanted to do something. You

know, she just had to do her job. And if I had just
laid there and had the baby and not let her stick
something in me or whatever, she just wasn't going to
be satisfied!

When I first got there and I dressed and everything she
wanted to give me an enema and I had been running
to the *bath*room all *morn*ing. I said lady (*high, incredu-*
lous), "There's none for you to wash *out!*" I said, "I
don't *need* an enema, I've been going to the bathroom
all morning!" (*conning the nurse in a whiney drawl*):
"Well you know, when you puuush that baaaby out,
ehhverythin' else is going to come out too—" I said,
(*in a mock black dialect*) "well huhhney, don't worry, I
don't think anything but a *baby* will come out and
getcha" (*laughing*):

She was just disgusted to no end—

(*clears throat*) and

so later on

I was doing *fine* and she—but the only thing is, because
I *didn't* eat

I was starting to feel nauseous and it, it was just the
kind of nausea feeling that you feel when you're
*hun*gry.

And I told her, I said, "I'm feeling a little sick on my
stomach, I haven't eaten anything all day" and I didn't
want to start heaving you know.

And so she said, "Well I can give you something for
that," and I said "Well *fine*, I'll *take* that."

And I didn't realize—I should have known: if it's
something to stop

your stomach from

doing that

it's going to be a muscle relaxer . . .

but at that time of

the *day* you're not thinking

and I just didn't want to start, you know, heaving like
that 'cause I wanted to

*con*centrate and I don't like to throw up—I get real
panicky—

and I thought the last thing I need is to start doing that.

So I agreed to *take* that.
And so she gave me that and then she said,
"Well, do you want anything for pain"? And I said,
  "Well, I don't really think so,
I'm doing all right." And she said, "Well if you *want*
something you're going to have to take it (*mock drawl*)
  nahw or it's not gonna work!"
By then I'm like, she's bein' a
bitch (*laughs*) you know and I'm like, just *whatever*
  (*laughs*)! Just (*high, emphatic*) leave me a*lone*! What
  will it take to make you go away? if you
give me something will you go away? So I think she,
  you know, gave me
some Demerol on top of this
. . . Once that kicked in?
I was no good.

I just, my head went back and it was like, OK, we can
  have a baby any time, you
know I don't care. Once that happened I just, I was not
  pushing. I didn't
feel—I couldn't really feel the contractions, they were
  having to tell me,
you're having a contraction now and you need to push
and, it just—
it went downhill from there.

I wasn't happy any more, and you can see on my pictures
  that I'm like
in a daze from all that medicine she had given me.
Even my doctor got mad at her.
Because, uh I mean like he was like, trying to *talk* to me
  and I'm just like
(*exhales*)
who are YOU? (*both laugh*)
I mean, I knew he was there and everything but I
  didn't care!
And he was like, "*What did you* . . . " I could hear him
talking to the nurse—

it's like I was,
almost like I was
in this little cage, and he was like, "*What did you GIVE her?*"
I had lost touch with my body by then.
And so, I was doing what Robert and the nurses and
the doctor were telling me to do . . .

—SAUNDRA[35]

It is errant, transgressive, sexy:

When it was *really* painful, it helped. . . back pressure
  helped. And
it was kind of funny because I kept (*laughing*) telling
  Mark, because it kept
getting worse and worse and I was like
  (*mocking orgasm*):
"*harder*, harder" and (*laughing*) Mark's leaning on me
  with *all* of
his weight (*laughs*). He's like, "Janet I don't think I can
  do it any—"
and I'd be like "HARDER, just tell me you're doing it
  harder!"
(*laughs*) He was like, "OK, OK, OK." Or I'd be
  like, like
as soon as I would . . . get into . . . really intense pain I
  would . . .
turn over on . . . all fours—this was toward the end
  when I was in
transition. And I would be like (*panting*):
"GET MY BACK GET MY BACK GET MY BACK"
  (*laughs*).
And he would just be like, "OK, OK!" I'd be like, "*lower*,
LOWER, LOWER!" And he'd go lower and I'd be like,
  "YES.
YES. HARDER—HARDER," like that (*laughs*). And
  he'd be
"OK!"
And it was just so funny.

—JANET[36]

It is desire un/fulfilled:

> I don't remember if it was before the first epidural
>   or not
>
> I know I was heavily into transition and
> I wasn't able—the contractions started and it was so
>   much more intense than any of the contractions
>   before it
> that I, I couldn't get, I couldn't breathe. I tried to
>   breathe and I couldn't breathe.
> You know and my eyes just started to tear, and it was
>   just like
> all I could do—I could feel this scream, and it was
> coming and my husband, I just I looked at my husband
>   and I saw this look
> on his face.
>
> This part always makes me cry, it's like
>
> (*crying*): it was like he couldn't help me
> you know, he was just desperate
> but he couldn't help me.
> He was just pleading with me to breathe, *just breathe,*
>   just breathe
> and he started doing the breathing for me so that
>   I could
> follow him. But that look on his face was just—
> there was just so much love there, and it just snapped
>   me out of this,
> this thing. You know, it snapped me out of my, my fear
>   and my panic
> it just knocked me out and I could breathe with him.
>
> It was the most touching part of the whole labor *really.*
>   It was that moment between the two of us, you
>   know, it was just incredible (*crying, laughing*).
>
>   —SUE[37]

It is beyond control:

> obviously the pain of childbirth is no fun, but
> um, it's a good kind of pain, ya know that it's
> producing something,
> ya know there's something happening that's a positive
> . . . event,
> and it's not pain from illness or something,
> but I think we've been trained to think of pain as
> something negative,
> so that women are afraid of it, you don't really talk
> about the pain.
> You say, Oh my labor was this long, and somebody
> might say, Yeah, when it really kicked in, or some-
> thing—
> but I found it was the thing most people were
> terrified of,
> and I was *surprised* that the one Lamaze class where
> that came out, a lot,
> once one woman said, I'm really scared how much this
> is gonna hurt, a lot of other people said, Yeah, and
> kinda, ya know pounced on that
> Yeah, like they were embarrassed to say that they were
> really afraid of it.
> But, I was surprised at the intensity of that fear,
> maybe because I'm able to talk to my husband about
> fears like that,
> I said, ya know, it's hard to know what to expect and
> how I'm going to respond to it,
> and the other thing is I guess that, we're both really
> strong in our Christian faith and I just felt kinda like,
> it's gonna go like it's gonna go, and we're gonna do our
> best and we've done all we can during the pregnancy,
> I've eaten well and exercised and all that,
> And, um, I just felt like, we've done our part and it's in
> God's hands,
> ya know, there's only so much worrying I can do about it,
> so we were fairly calm about the whole thing,

and whatever comes, we'll deal with it somehow,
and when I heard these other women who were,
who were having nightmares, who, ya know were almost
 shaking even talking about being so afraid of the pain,
I thought, Wow, ya know, that was something I
 didn't share,
and I'm glad I didn't.

I come back to the idea of the religious side of it, too—
I'm not the kind of Christian who goes around, ya
 know, shoving pamphlets down people's throats, that
 kind of thing,
so I hadn't really mentioned it to the midwife or
 anything,
but she had said to me that
she was surprised that women who do feel strongly
 about their religion, not any particular one, seemed to
 have an easier time in labor and delivery,
because they were able to let go, they didn't feel as much
 of a need to be in absolute control of themselves.

        —CHARLOTTE[38]

It is grievous:

I can remember having a doctor tell me when I was
when I was weeping, like a week after
losing
one
pregnancy
I had to go back in for a second D&C (dilatation and
 curettage), and of course they're painful in the first
 place.
And, and *habitually* there's inadequate . . . painkiller . . .
 given . . .
for a D&C. I mean it's . . .
If a *man* were having such procedure done, I am
 *ab*solutely *po*sitive it wouldn't be done under the same
 circumstances. I'm just positive it wouldn't.
And ah . . .

so there I
was lying there, having a D&C done, and
the tears . . . going down my cheeks, and the doctor
    said, "You know I really . . . think you . . . ought to
    consider seeing somebody" (which I was anyway, I
    had been since I'd lost the first baby).
He said, "You know you . . . you really are experiencing
    what I
think is un*na*tural grief."
Unnatural grief—(*ironic, wistful*) a full week
after losing a
three-month pregnancy.

After the second miscarriage I think
I ceased thinking of pregnancy as . . . something that led
    to a child anymore. I started thinking of pregnancy as
    something that led to grief and distraction.
I knew very *well* in my conscious mind that thinking in
    that way didn't protect me from the grief when it
    happened.
All you do then is suffer it ahead of time and suffer it
    again when it happens—it doesn't protect you at *all* to
    suffer it ahead of time. You might as well be hopeful
    and optimistic, at least you get the benefit of *that* . . .
    until you get—crushed.

But I just couldn't . . .
I said to Ken
that until the day after the twins were born,
I never believed deep in my heart that they would
be born.
I never believed it.
I really didn't.
I still look at them and think, where did you
    come from?
You know?
Where on *earth* did you come from?

        —DEBORAH[39]

Deborah's story ends with the grown-up version of the child's plea, where did I/where do babies come from? *Where did you come from?* she asks, turning the question back on the child. Her story rises to the question with which so many others begin, suggesting that even in this double birth, coming as it did after five miscarriages, she is bereft of an origin, of an anchor in a world rife with loss. Lacking now either a proper beginning or end, Deborah's story, like Margaret's and others', was a story of memory, of the power of pain to write its own story and to make experience answer to its memory. The memory of pain keeps Deborah's story and life, her storied life and life stories, open, ragged, so weary with crushed hopes that hope itself seems false. Deborah's obstetrician was concerned about what he called the "unnatural" length of her grief one week after her second miscarriage. Should the pain have gone away? Should it, could it have been unremembered—and her body/imagination freed to pursue happier ends? What story was Deborah supposed to tell that, remembering the pain of five miscarriages, she "failed" to tell?

Where did you come from? The twins were born in pain. Deborah bore the twins and pain. Her story reflects their shared origin in miscarriage, underscored as it was by grief, loss, a sense of having failed norms of medicine and maternity, of her body having failed her. Had she not remembered her miscarriages as acutely as she did, she might have told a different story. A much less ambivalent story, a story founded—originating—in desire without lack. Deborah was effectively chastised for, in miscarrying, diverging from preferred, medical/ized narratives of "successful" pregnancies and limited grief, for remembering pain in life/story performance. But what or whose story would she tell without the memory of pain? Would she have a story without remembered pain? Conversely, is there pain without memory? Is pain what it is because it is remembered—and therefore nothing when it's not?[40]

To take the question one step further: if pain lives in its subjective/symbolic value, in the stories memory writes, where is it (is it?) when narrative either fails or is presumed to fail? The question itself tends to privilege neurological pain. It positions pain as an object of memory, a thing to be remembered, and hence fundamentally separate from and prior to the cognitive capacity for symbol making. As such, it writes pain painless in figures of a pre- or postsymbolic life, figures considered neurologically or symbolically immature—animals and old people and infants, for instance, who might then be ignored or left crying, or African Americans whose slave ancestors, considered by their master/owners to be half-animal, were beaten savagely, as if in order for the beating to be "meaningful" within the disciplinary structure of a slave economy it had to make up in savagery for the slave's alleged lack of human feeling and wit.[41] Modern psychoanalytics moreover tend to dismiss as hysterical women whose narratives seem to fail them by failing standards of normal/normative discourse, who do not relate their pain within familiar or "appropriate" forms for memory. Unformed or, for all intents and purposes, linguistically deformed, their pain must be (or so the story goes) phantasmic.[42]

Identifying pain with memory and narrative thus has often been used against those whose difference marks them outside, beyond, or threatening to the given discursive order. In this light it is tempting to say that pain is pain: that it cuts across class, race, age, gender, and species, leveling hierarchy in the commonality of sensate life. But to do so, at least in the context of thinking about birth stories, is to conspire with those discourses that dismiss or effectively retire birth pain, often in the name of so-called maternal amnesia. Folk discourses of amnesia (sometimes attributed to the postpartum rush of prolactin, a relaxing hormone, stimulated by nursing) tend to reserve the language of pain for labor pain, to bracket off other dimensions of the birth experience from identification with pain, and to render both (the latter already subordinated to the former) speechless or forgotten as pain to speech. They cast pain as essential/universal and, as such, make it forgettable (it is prediscursive, prememory). Hence, many of the stories I heard were punctuated with apologies for what had been, in effect, forbidden to memory: *You forget . . . I've forgotten . . . I can't really remember the pain but I remember . . .*

Hence, too, drugs may be overprescribed for birth, as they were for Saundra, and, as Deborah noted, underprescribed for dilatation and curettage, or "D&C," the procedure routinely performed after miscarriage to remove any residual embryonic tissue from the uterus, in Saundra's case, short-circuiting pain that was beginning to feel like power and, in Deborah's case, underscoring by ignoring the pain that then signified her "failure" to have carried a fetus to term. Accordingly, Saundra's pain became the pain of forced forgetting, Deborah's of being pointedly forgotten to discourses of "successful" pregnancies. In both cases pain and forgetting were linked in discipline, in making the prospective mother conform to norms of compliance and reproduction, to become a mother defined at once by identification with and transcendence of birth pain. In other words, at least in these cases pain was not forgotten at all but transmuted into social effects, and memory was not the prerogative of the individual, for whom physical pain may or may not remain a conscious token of experience, but was itself social and collective. Remembering their respective and multiple versions of pain, Saundra and Deborah felt themselves remembered to pain: positioned within discourses of pain, pain management, and maternity for which their bodies became a kind of proof. They felt themselves written by pain (or the instituted lack thereof) into a story that was far larger than either of them, that exceeded individual control, and that would, it seemed, reproduce itself in a long genealogy of their own and others' "experience."[43]

Birth stories occur in the time neither of memory nor of myth nor of remembered pain. They occur in the time of remembering, in the passage from memory to recall to reflexivity and remaking. They emerge in the space between a teller and a listener, belonging to neither, changing by the moment, by the moment-to-moment play of conversational perspectives, and by context—so that most of the stories I heard from women and men I knew primarily through participation in prenatal classes echoed the form and perspective of the medical narratives we'd heard there, and a friend noted after two hours of conversation, embarrassed, "I should have asked which of the hundred stories you wanted to hear!" Birth stories shift, sediment, change over time, so that the story I tell of Isabel's birth now has more to do with her subsequent care in the neonatal intensive care unit than with, as it did for years, our confrontation with hospital birthing routines and, in a much shorter time, one woman's story shifted from the plane of metaphorical reflection on which she told her story to me to the kind of blow-by-blow plotting with which she and the five other members of her "new moms" group drew each other into transgressive revelry. Ordinary, in time, practicing the life and politics of the body in various (patient, strained, loving, erotic) relations to other bodies, other lives, no one of these stories is more "true" than another. All reflect the ordinary truth of many truths, sometimes divided against each other, sometimes conjoined, like desire and loss, in the paradoxical expression of pain.

Birth stories belong to the time of re/membering. Contingent on time, they are nonetheless as story-performances, as stories emerging, unfolding, cresting and breaking in time, of and about time. They constitute performative "contact zones," drawing narrator and listener into, at once, contact with each other and, through each other, with the broader cultural narratives their respective performances enact and challenge.[44] Performed *in relation to*, in reciprocal engagement with a listener, a friend, an imagined community, an institution crowding in on the very body of the story, the stories enter time through address, in flashing reference to the "other" whose otherness underwrites the act of telling, anticipating its turns with its own and turning again in turn. Under the backwash of otherness, the story/subject becomes other to itself/herself, un/knowing itself in reflexivity, under pressure of a kind of self/other-witnessing that propels the/a story forward, into dialogic relation with itself as an other, into the obscene im/possibility of what the literary theorist Mikhail Bakhtin has called an "eternal" becoming (Bakhtin 1984a:252). Underscored by the peculiar intensities of reflexivity, mobilized by time into time (rather than, say, mythic timelessness or distant memory) through the ordinary embodied practice of remembering, refiguring pain in the image of present and future social, symbolic relations and so re/marking its ordinariness, making it—against the pressure of forgetting and silence and dull surrender to unconscious routine—remarkable: birth stories bring pain into an open field of representation—and let it loose.

CHAPTER FOUR

Secrets/Doubles

Having learned the habit of hiding, I found I had also learned to hide from myself. I did not know who I was, only that I did not want to be they, the ones who are destroyed or dismissed to make the "real" people, the important people, feel safer. . . . Hide, hide to survive, I thought, knowing that if I told the truth about my life, my family, my sexual desire, my history, I would move over into that unknown territory, the land of they, would never have a chance to name my own life, to understand it or to claim it.

—Dorothy Allison, "A Question of Class"

I must make the final gesture of defiance, and refuse to let this be absorbed by the central story; must ask for a structure of political thought that will take all of this, all these secret and impossible stories, recognize what has been made out on the margins; and then, recognizing it, refuse to celebrate it; a politics that will, watching this past say "So what?"; and consign it to the dark.

—Carolyn Steedman, *Landscape for a Good Woman*

A SECRET EXISTS in performative relation to its other, its mirror double: exposure, explicitness. Secrecy marks a border; it is a border space, a play space, whose simplest pleasures are enacted in the child's game of "making up" secrets. The child's secret is meant to be told, to be passed in eartight talk back and forth, from one person to the next. The pleasure of playing "telephone," for instance, lies in hearing secrets travel the byways of memory and imagination, accumulating disorder as they cross from one body context to another, twisting and transforming in the play of private public knowledge or the construction of what we call rumors.[1]

Language is secretive. It keeps secrets, keeps truths, or keeps truths secret, hidden in the folds of representational practice. Inseparable from the means by which it is conveyed, truth is the secret language keeps. In the performance of secrecy language reveals how it conceals, how it operates in worlds we think we know because we recognize their representational forms—but where, in fact, mis/recognition rules. As Peggy Phelan (1993:2–3) has argued, "the real is read through representation, and representation is read through the real." What we see may snow-blind us to the fact that what we see—the "visible real"—is the truth effect of discursive, representational or, in the end, decoy realities.[2]

Language is fickle (Bakhtin 1984a:202). It betrays its origins in a particular speech context even as it passes from that context to another. Always already slipping from one social code into the arms of another (mixing their scents and sense), any single utterance is divided, double-voiced, inflected at least twice over by the difference between competing claims on what it does or should mean.

Understood as a mobile and elusive grammar of social relations, language is epitomized in rumors and gossip, the very stuff of social knowledge. While *faking* and practices of *truth taking* (often literally charging subjects with shamming and lying in order to depose, discover, uncover the truth)[3] have conventionally defined the realm of the secret, *truth making* shifts the register of accountability from truth to knowledge, from the absolutist plane of *finding truth* to the shabbier social practice of *making knowledge*.[4] What I heard, what you heard—these are the grounds of local knowledge.

As a social, performative practice, secrecy confers and maintains identities, distinguishing insiders (those in the know) from outsiders. It defines circles of knowledge, enabling alternative sites of social knowledge production to emerge and thrive. As Allen Feldman has observed:

> In a colonized culture, secrecy is an assertion of identity and of symbolic capital. Pushed to the margins, subaltern groups construct their own margins as fragile insulations from the "center." Secrecy is the creation of centers in peripheries deprived of stable anchorages.
> (FELDMAN 1991:11)

Secrecy constructs the borders it guards. It is the place where knowing and not knowing divide—but it is also the place where disguise and surveillance meet.[5] Secrecy may be a group's last or only defense against incursion and imperialization.[6] It may protect not only ideas and information but the lives of those who keep them. It requires, commands vigilance. But, in the end, secrecy can provide only, as Feldman notes, "fragile" insulation and remains a borderland of "unknowing," mis/representation, improvisation, and the occasional magic of masquerade.

∗ ∗ ∗ ∗

We live in a tabloid culture. The slow build to trust among friends, the pregnant pause (!) now seem as old-fashioned as black and white family "snaps" and pages turned out on a typewriter. Talk has fallen away against the rise of the talk show: the spectacle of disclosure, the supersimulation of experience and identity, the sensational production of "raw" feelings— all have made the TV confessional into the model of contemporary discourse.[7]

Talk show talk doesn't dispense with distinctions between what's public and what's private as much as it fetishizes privacy in the public realm. It makes what's private public not only by putting up for display and consumption every detail of lived lives but by producing those lives accordingly. The lives rehearsed in prime-time are subject to expert analysis, hyperpathology (I'm OK, you're OK seems to have been replaced by I'm in recovery, you're in denial), and standards of dramatic appeal that, above all, curtail reflection on the politics of subjectivity. Talk shows pin identity to an apparently endless run on sound bites (women who hate men, men who hate women, women who love men who hate women, etc.) and literally create lives in the fantastical reunion of, for instance, birth mothers and adopted children or forced confrontations between "children and the parents who left them." It is no surprise that much of the talk show phenomenon is devoted to the admission and construction of sexual histories. Where it departs from the explicit review of sexual lives, in the form of the political call-in show or the late-night interview show, for instance, or in the larger spectacles of the Clarence Thomas hearings and the O. J. Simpson trial, it tends to sublimate direct sexual appeal in political and celebrity frenzy.

In all of these ways and more talk show discourse makes life seem delectably transparent. It gives the impression that there is nothing left to know and nothing worth knowing that isn't already made known within the tight frame of the studio camera and lapel mike. By the codes of talk show talk: there is, happily, nothing left to hide.

I agree that, as Kenneth Plummer has argued, "stories of the body need to be told, especially, that will connect it to *reproduction* (reproductive politics, abortion, reproductive rights, pregnancy, genetic engineering and all the new technologies of reproduction)" (Plummer 1995:157). As I have tried to show throughout these pages, stories are templates for action and identity. They are sites of reflection, critique, self-making, self-theorizing, and collectivization.[8] They are inventions on memory, the substance of cogenerative, regenerative play. As such, they hold out the prospect of deepened intimacies, even an erotics of everyday life.

But I am leery of the extent to which, in the rush to story, we leave behind the power of the secret or, more to the point, of secrecy: the power of performing at the threshold of knowing and not-knowing, of producing opacities and ambiguities in the place of spectacular transparencies, of refusing subordination to surveillant technocracies not by hiding out exactly but by hiding *out*, in the open: by making secrecy, although not necessarily secret information, known.

In this light I want to rethink "the secret" not as an object of revelation but as a boundary phenomenon, as the visible figure of an elusive unknown. Understood in this way, silence is not there to be broken (as the strange alliance of some feminist and TV/consumerist discourses might suggest). Silence around birth and maternity may indeed be dangerous (Chesler 1979:62). But *breaking* silence may be equally if not more so. It may reiterate the violence that often produces silence in the first place. It threatens protective silence—the silence in which, for instance, Dorothy Allison hid in order to avoid being "destroyed or dismissed," the silence in which she found at least provisional safety. Breaking silence, telling intimate stories, may become compulsive (even in light of Steedman's sense of the "compulsions of narrative"); it may become subject to feminist and/or Jerry Springer norms that suggest silence is bad, perverse, even pathological, anticipating full assimilation to the disciplinary ethic of an *exposé* culture: tell all, come clean.[9]

Within this cultural milieu secrets are dirty. Dirty little secrets. Telling secrets may reproduce discourses of shame, embarrassment, and domination.[10] Performing secrecy, to the contrary, makes tacit claims on confidentiality. It seduces the listener into obligation to keep the secret secret, to linger (more gatekeeper than trespasser) on the tenuous line between knowing and not knowing, enjoying the likelihood of never knowing, of keeping what's not known *unknown*, marking the performative power of secrecy with vague allusions and masked identities. It refuses to let secret, taboo, impossible stories be "absorbed by the central story," not by rehearsing taboos but by denying rights of access and demanding, implicitly or explicitly, an alternative "structure of political thought that will take all of this, all these secret and impossible stories, recognize what has been made out on the margins; and then, recognizing it, refuse to celebrate it," a politics that will neither dismiss nor idealize the secret, preferring instead the power of refusal, the protocols of reserve and the retributions of darkness.

In this light, I want to echo D. A. Miller's (1977:207) sense that

in a world where the explicit exposure of the subject would manifest how thoroughly he [*sic*] has been inscribed within a given social totality, secrecy would be the spiritual exercise by which the subject is allowed to conceive of himself as a resistance: as a friction in the smooth functioning of the social order, a margin to which its far-reaching discourse does not reach.

Performing secrecy sustains a difference between public worlds and private selves. It recovers "phantasmatic" oppositions between private and public, inside and outside, subject and object, that tremble under the weight of revelation and disclosure. Making public knowledge secret, making privacy public: *performing secrecy* appropriates binarisms that have for so long kept women private, inside, and suspect. It turns the secret inside out, composing what Miller calls "open secrets." For Miller, "We know perfectly well that the secret is known, but nonetheless we must persist, however ineptly, in guarding it": "The paradox of the open secret registers the subject's accommodation to a totalizing system that has obliterated the difference he would make—the difference he does make, in the imaginary denial of this system, 'even so.'" Secrets bear the signs of subjection. Recalling public knowledge to secrecy (as Steedman does, for instance) or telling secrets *secretly* resists the subjection secrets tell. Performing secrecy, even by resurrecting false oppositions between public and private, inside and outside, in an "imaginary denial" of total subjection, repositions the self as *resistance*, as "a friction in the smooth functioning of the social order." As the guardian of secret ways, the self may or may not bare the secrets she carries. She wields silence. She makes a difference by marking a difference between what she knows and what she may tell, making her listener subject to the hushed or brazen pleasures of her own secret ways.

In the course of talking with people about birth I often felt myself *subject to* secrets, drawn into hiding, recruited into compliance with their particular ethics and politics. I participated in these, among other, *secret scenes:*

I.

I talked with Jaylin, a prenatal instructor at a large teaching hospital, through a veil of household duties. She tried to get her nine-month old to eat a little cold soup before her husband, Carl, returned with the truck, keeping her eye all the while on their two-year-old son playing relentlessly on the stairs, messing up what she kept straightening up. They were trying to get away for the weekend. Shortly after Carl arrived, I packed up my things, wanting to get out of their way; Jaylin walked me to my car. As we crossed from the stairs of her apartment unit to the parking lot, catching the sudden glare of a high, hot sun, she looked around, apparently checking to see who might see or hear us. Still looking out but confident, it seemed, that no one was within earshot, she told me what she apparently couldn't when we were inside, where her husband and two boys were never more than a few feet away. Stumbling slightly, wavering between saying and not saying, between hoping to be and not having been heard, she offered this aside to our recorded conversation: It's good you are doing this. There are a lot of women who need *(her voice dropping, catching)* to tell what happened.[11]

2.

Doug sat in front of me, Randy by my side, both relaying the pleasure they'd taken in joking around with their obstetrician, the nurses, even the anesthesiologist who administered the epidural. It was a relief, they explained, the birth was "fun." *I took up their pleasure instantly, laughing along with the absurdities of a doctor on his third day of call and the speed with which everything—baby, placenta,* "everything"—"just kind of shot right out." *Doug watched Randy deal with chronic pain daily. He consequently wanted the birth to be as painless as possible. He quickly shed the machismo he associated with the pain of a "natural" childbirth:* "When they say that some guys mind if the wife does that, they want them to have natural, I just, I, you know, I couldn't imagine." *This too became a joke. Once, Doug said, the doctor came into their room trailing the sounds of a woman down the hall screaming her lungs out . . .* "Is she taking drugs?" *Randy had asked.* "No, but I wish she would!" *the doctor had answered—with mock anger to general laughter.*

But Doug *still seemed to feel compelled to defend his son's birth against invisible lurking charges that it wasn't "natural." Randy had had, as Doug put it,* "everything"—*external and internal fetal monitors, epidural, episiotomy—all relatively routine measures of a hospital birth. He justified the epidural by sympathy with Randy's pain; he legitimized the episiotomy by reference to secret medical knowledge (more sure, it seemed, for being secret); leaning in, he told me what the doctor told them. He asked,* "You know what he told us?" *I didn't, of course, expecting another punchline:*

"He said, 'I'm not being prejudiced, but you know that ninety percent of all white women have to have [an] episiotomy, and ninety percent of all black women don't.'

He said, 'Ninety percent of most white women tear. And the black women don't.'

He said, 'I don't have any idea why, and I won't say that around anybody 'cause they'll say that I'm . . . prejudiced or something about it.'

'But,' he said, 'But I've done this for years and . . .'

He said, 'I give episiotomies to almost all white ladies but very, very few black ladies need it.'"

"Isn't that wild?" *Doug concluded. I answered back with another question, weakly confirming Doug's trust in me and the doctor, and the doctor's trust in him, deferring all questions of race to Doug's confidence in the doctor's acquired wisdom, which, reiterated as it was in Doug's litany of quotations, suggested that an episiotomy was in fact "natural" for white women. I secured the suggestion with a question that, for all intents and purposes, closed the doctor's logic;* "So, he's really doing it on the basis of need?" *I wasn't just "anybody" now; I was in on what the doctor wouldn't say around just "anybody." I was a white lady who'd torn and ripped and been cut and sewn and who'd been trusted, as were Doug and Randy, through Doug and Randy, not to challenge the doctor's race-based logic, to keep the secret between us, not to "say . . . something about it." I performed accordingly—until now.*[12]

3.

An old college friend, Elyse, recorded this exchange among the members of her "new moms" group in Chicago; I listened in weeks and miles away. I did more than eavesdrop really. I had the tape, I owned it. I played and replayed it, playing the very Oprah-watching, scandal-mongering voyeur they parodied:

LAURIE: So I went in the shower and then ahhhm, it was funny
I'd forgotten: I *shit* in the shower.
And I totally blocked that out. And it was like,
I can remember being in the shower, being totally

conscious of oh my God I have to go the bathroom.
I'm in the middle of a contraction and I can't do both
at once (*laughter*).

I can only focus on getting through the contraction and
I couldn't focus on getting through the contraction
and getting out of the shower (*laughter*) and going to
the bathroom, you know. So I just shit in the shower.
I just like—

and then I remember laughing going, "Manny, I just shit
in the shower."

He's like, "Oh that's OK." I mean you'd think he'd spent
his whole life cleaning bed pans and stuff (*laughter*).

"I'll clean it up . . . ," you know, I'm sure it was like so
gross

but he just did it, you know (*laughter*).

The next thing I know I'm back in the shower. Then I
was kind of relieved

because I'd rather do *it* at my house, you know.

I heard, I heard that on *Oprah* once, you know.

ELYSE: I heard that on *Oprah*, too.

LAURIE: *"Horrible stories of where you hide your shit during
            your labor!"*

DIANNE: Oh wait a minute, Oprah did a special show on that . . .
            *"Did you shit in the shower during your labor?
            Call 1–800- . . . !"* (*general laughter*).[13]

✳ ✳ ✳ ✳

Need.
Untold desire. Un/desire. Depression.
Race.
Shit.
Laughter.
Dirty little secrets. Underworlds. Underwords. Made public, in confidence. Under/excessively represented.
Slips. Asides.

    Secrets circulated throughout the interview process. Confessed, deployed, forgotten/remembered—they broke the boundaries of public/private life. Secrecy—the hushed tone of Jaylin's half-confession, the sense of being in the know I shared with Doug and Randy, the new moms' members-only joke on what it might mean to make shit *spectacular*—bridged the double spaces secrets traversed. A secret is a secret because it is not/could be public knowledge. It is disclosed only *within* a circle of declared membership or as a means of *drawing in* the outsider, producing membership, for instance, in an alliance of whiteness and medical authority, or told *inside-out*, when what's usually "outside"—husband, work, weekend plans—has rushed in and driven the secret *out*. With Carl's return Jaylin's apartment had suddenly become both too personal and too public. Outside, in the parking lot, her secret belonged to everyone and to no one, to "a lot of women"—not Jaylin, not me, not just her, not just me. Secrets may be so personal that they are forgotten, repressed, blocked (like shitting during childbirth) or heralded on prime-time TV: they are a taboo memory on the verge of becoming a taboo sensation. A secret may be, as it was in Elyse's moms' group, performed *outside-in*: official knowledge and privileged ways of knowing may be brought into the folds of private parody, generating a "hidden transcript" about to burst at the seams.[14]

The secret is itself two-faced. As a secret, embedded in *secrecy*, it double talks, permeating the delicate membranes that keep inside from out. It is twice powerful: as a mask and in the performativity of *unmasking*—not revealing a hidden truth as much as the mask that hides it. It is double(d) in the precarious possibility of *telling*. Whispered, half-told, announced, secrets unfold as both *risk* and *power*: as the risk of embarrassment, shame, helplessness, betrayal, and judgment, and as the power of knowledge and (cabbalistic) authority.

What does it mean for me to tell these secrets now? What did it mean for me to hear them, to participate in the particular circles of secrecy they drew? There was a perverse intimacy in each of these scenes—an intimacy bound to renewing given political structures by rehearsing prohibitions against body *knowing*. Jaylin admitted her error, fault, need. Doug and Randy, encouraged by their doctor's lead, othered Southern women and black women (performed their difference as deviance) in bad jokes and statistical review. Elyse and her friends dramatized the media marketing of forbidden bodies. All deferred authority—to what "a lot of women" need, what the doctor knows, what Oprah wants.[15] Each conversation more or less reinforced race, class, sex, gender hierarchies. In each I complied with bans on certain bodies (bodies in pain, excremental bodies, black female bodies). And yet each also retained a trace, a promise of something else. *Telling* proved excessive. It filled and spilled over confession, bad jokes and expertise in hilarity, intensity, asides. It blurred bodies and bodies of knowledge in feeling that was nevertheless just as quickly written over by narratives in which women are wrong, doctors are right, and bad is, however seductively, bad. Telling secret stories did not in itself make a difference. And yet, in sudden gasps, it promised what Plummer (1995) has called "intimate citizenship": a deepened sense of self and community built on telling untold, banned, withheld stories, not on making private worlds public so much as refusing exclusion by privatization. I proceeded on this promise and yet often felt burdened by secrets—unwilling to keep them, unable to *bear* them, unable not to.[16]

Walking out on the hot asphalt with Jaylin, listening to her commend my project with implicit thanks for answering her own "need," for providing a space in which she could admit at once to what she called her "failure" to manage pain appropriately, to exemplify the methodical composure she taught her students weekly, and to the crazy power she felt in putting off pushing until her mother arrived much later, I suddenly felt clammy, cold. Would I be the confessor to other women's secret needs, needs they keep secret even from themselves? Was Jaylin authorizing me, in her capacity as a prenatal instructor, to pick up the pieces, to recuperate both shame and transgressive joy to the official narratives she taught? Here, outside her home, at the edges of the cold soup/weekend trip world to which her waiting family called her, I felt drawn into a secret pact: to recognize and respond to other women's secret need to tell, to be heard, to feel confirmed in their deviance from *the* story under cover of "research." Suddenly any other dimension of the project seemed secondary to what Jaylin assumed we both knew: that this was the real, the secret, the true reason I was out and about. That the unspoken rule to which we both answered was solace, consolation. But keep the secret secret, she seemed to say. Don't let anyone know. Watch out. Don't tell what we both know but won't say except in this short slant moment. I got into my car. Felt the smile I offered in sympathy and gratitude begin to crack. Found the air conditioning and drove away.

****

Hiding in the Open

Ruth was a student in one of my performance studies classes.[17] She attended class irregularly for the first three or four weeks, rarely speaking during that time, except in a performance that required students to reflect on their family histories. She mesmerized the class with an account of visiting her aunt and eight cousins at the family homeplace. Her voice suddenly deep and wide, she drew us into her origins in place and play: "In the front yard there were these two huge pecan trees," she said, "that were rooted on each side of the sidewalk that led up to the front porch. These trees were ideal for climbing and imaginary tree houses. We used to pretend that the trees were our houses so we all divided up into three families of mamas, daddies, and chaps. This was convenient because there were only three boys and the rest of us were girls. We tried to disguise our game because the adults didn't believe in kinfolk playing such mama and daddy games. We didn't care because we had so much fun playing that we didn't have time to think about what mamas and daddies did when they were away from their children. We were having so much fun that we didn't even want to stop playing to eat our dinner."[18]

I didn't know that Ruth was pregnant until we began to talk about the story, when she remarked that she would be the third of three generations of single mothers in her family, a family overrun by women (she hoped she'd have a boy). And then she disappeared. She was gone for five, six weeks, entirely out of contact, except by rumor that she was having her baby—and unreachable. Partly on my instigation, the class wanted to convey congratulations, to find out how she was. I tried her number again, and again, each long series of rings intensifying my desire to find her. I never did.

And then she reappeared in class one day, with a tiny baby in a car seat. She sat, as before, near the front, to the side. We cooed over the baby and satisfied our sense of protocol by presenting her with the baby present I'd been storing in my office, awaiting her return, bringing her into our circle of attention.

Her next performance, however, spun that circle hard. She began the performance sitting in silence in the center of the large room; we sat around her in a wide arc. She proceeded to bare her left, full breast and to nurse her baby while repeating the discourses that crossed through her and would have pulled her apart had she not, it seemed, assumed the full authority of her bodily presence, as she did now. While her first performance drew three generations into a single line of female strength, this one was split three and four ways into fragments of recrimination, demands, and defensiveness, all in a context that made the pecan trees and summer days of her first performance seem largely nostalgic. We now heard the voices of aunts, friends, Ruth, the baby's father criss-crossing in violent confusion but with a kind of epigrammatic clarity:

"Why don't you get her [the baby's] father to help you?"
"all them, no good, deadbeat dads"
"he bought those diapers"
"I got to look out for my other kids, too"

And then she was gone again. And again I felt the keen absence of her presence. She was always overwhelmingly *there* or *not there*. I consequently didn't know quite what to say when I ran into her sometime later in town, although I finally did ask whether she'd like to record her birth stories in conversation. She said she would—although I think at first out of a sense of bemused compliance.

We sat side by side in my office (her choice), with the tape recorder between us on the desk. I quickly summarized the project in light of some of the issues we had addressed in class, trying to find my footing, while she waited patiently, half-smiling—at my awkwardness? I wondered, or, as it turned out, in anticipation of performing secrecy, telling *secrets* only incidentally to conveying the strategies by which she passed through hospital bureaucracies: her secret means, her clever ruse. She'd mentioned having just petitioned social services for receipt of welfare benefits. I turned on the recorder and stumbled right to the point:

DELLA: What difference did it make to you
do you think, in the birth
or . . . around the birth
that—
your identity was in part African American and
tied to receiving
public funding, does that—?

RUTH: Well . . .
I think it would have affected me more had I not sort of
tricked the hospital.

DELLA: Really?

RUTH: Yeah. At one time I had medical insurance before
I became pregnant and before my mother quit her job
she had insurance on me and I sort of slipped that
insurance through the hospital, sort of as a—

DELLA: Oh . . .
So you t—you told them that's what . . . ?

RUTH: Yes. I gave them the insurance information knowing
that I did have Medicaid
only because I had seen how badly
my cousin had been treated when she was in
the hospital.[19]

Ruth "sort of tricked the hospital." She kept her current insurance status a secret. She "slipped through" an old card. But the trick turned not on what she concealed but on what, in concealing her insurance status, she revealed: that what passed for the rational administration of insurance identities was in fact crudely arbitrary and that class/race privilege is radically contingent. The hospital divided up its obstetric patients on the basis of their insurance status. Their insurance cards became the insignia of their bodies, their lives, their selves, which were then routed (private insurance, this way; Medicaid, that way) and treated accordingly. Ruth had seen, for instance, how her cousin's insurance card marked her for isolation and recrimination:

RUTH: [In the city where my cousin gave birth] they have a
policy where, if you're
on Medicaid, they room you with two people—
well, there's
two people to a room
and . . . you're considered "staff."
You're located on one side of the hospital which is
not so
nice and you don't have the birthing suites
um when you're on Medicaid.
DELLA: You're considered staff?
RUTH: Yes. You're called staff patients.
And I researched this before I came
to deliver Ifra at [a local hospital] because I didn't
want to
be looked down upon
DELLA: Yeah.
RUTH: because my cousin was a staff patient and I saw how
ugly she was treated
in the hospital. It's just because you have
a *label* placed upon you, "*staff*," because you have

> *Medicaid.* Which is a type of insurance that some
> people seem to overlook.
> DELLA: Right.
> RUTH: And, um, in her room
> it was her and another girl
> and . . . occasionally the nurses would come by
> and they would, you know, do their routine checks but
> they weren't very cordial
> they weren't greeting, they weren't very nice at all and I
> was saying, "Oh, my God, when I have my baby I
> just don't want to be *treated* like that."

Ruth's cousin's card positioned her within the hospital's power/knowledge matrix as a "staff patient." Being on the "staff ward" meant having both less privacy and less attention. It meant that her body was both more exposed and more vulnerable to various disciplinary measures. It was spectacularized for presumably sexual, moral excesses that were then contained by isolation to the ward and (at best) slighting regard.

On the warrant of her insurance card the hospital produced Ruth's cousin as a staff patient who basically deserved only and whatever she got. She became the relatively docile subject of the way the hospital practiced class distinctions or "the way things are around here." Ruth saw "the way things are" for what they were: the consolidation of routine procedures in a presumptive reality based on pinning the self to a sign of the self, fixing her cousin in the identity position her insurance card carved out for her.

At the time Ruth was on Medicaid. She indicated as much to the billing office upon discharge. But she got in on a recently expired insurance card, whether by luck of an oversight or some ambiguity in the card itself, and, in so doing, dramatized the slippery relation between the self and the sign-systems to which it is subject. Ruth tricked the trick. She saw through the hospital's discursive regime to the identity game it played—and trumped it.[20]

Plying her double/secret knowledge (knowing she had been and was not privately insured, knowing that the hospital's class bias was so deeply buried under the appearance of administrative rationality as to be practically imperceptible, even to those who enforced it), Ruth slipped the grip of the hospital's identity system. She produced ludic space in the place of easy class/race distinctions. She found the *play*, the elasticity, in what otherwise seems a fixed identity system, noting, among other things, how differently her cousin was treated when the nurses discovered that she was, in fact, *one of them*: that her mother worked for the hospital.

Suddenly, the outsider-inside became a legitimate insider: the nurses who "weren't very nice at all" were suddenly cordial and concerned. Which meant that Ruth saw her cousin and the nurses shift identity positions, revealing spaces between identities, between selves and signs of the self, and among the mobile, partial, contingent identities she consequently saw herself playing.

Ruth reveled in her "ingenious plan," arguing that "I've noticed that when I used my Medicaid card before having Ifra with getting prescriptions and for just medical expenses, you're treated really differently." Ruth insists that "insurance is insurance." Insurance means insurance. It is a self-same signifier. It doesn't signify the identity differences it is nonetheless used to produce:

DELLA:	How are you treated differently?
RUTH:	OK. Um . . .
	for example, all right, I had Blue Cross and Blue Shield at one time.
	And . . . later, I—of course, I got my Medicaid once the insurance policy
	lapsed or whatever
	and I would take my—you know as long as I had my co-pay card, they would gladly accept that, and I was greeted and treated very nice.
	Almost as if I—
	I was somebody important.
	However I've noticed when I took my *Medicaid* card they sort of
	you know, snatched the card from me and
	if there was any additional information that
	they needed
	they would
	ask for it as if I couldn't answer the question . . .
DELLA:	Ohh . . .
RUTH:	as well as I might have been able to. And it—I really felt sort of
	displaced, I felt embarrassed. I felt
	real, I felt really small.
	Really small.
DELLA:	I bet.
RUTH:	And . . . I don't think that it should make a difference

whether you're an insured patient with Blue Cross or
Kaiser Permanente or whoever
because, I don't know, insurance is insurance to me.

DELLA: Yeah.

RUTH: And I noticed that recently—this happened
just not too long ago—um, I went in
to see Ifra's doctor
and um . . . automatically—

Now, mind you, there were other patients in front of
me. There was
particularly a white lady in front of me
who *had* Medicaid.
But the lady—um, the receptionist asked her
about her insurance status. She was like, "Who are
you insured by?" and she [the woman in line] gave
her her Medicaid card. She [the receptionist]
didn't say anything else. But when it came to *me*
she says (*loud voice*):
"Um, do you have your Medicaid card with
you today?"
As if
I couldn't have insurance or wouldn't be insured by . . .
a company per se.
And that really made me, you know, sort of look at that
situation because who was—I mean, you couldn't tell
the difference: I was dressed nicely and the lady in
front of me she—looked about equivalent to me
and the receptionist didn't ask *her* for a Medicaid card,
but she automatically assumed that I was on Medicaid, and there's no
indications on Ifra's record that she was on Medicaid
because this was a new doctor that she was going to.

DELLA: So what—what kind of assumptions
was she making
then?

RUTH: Well . . .
well in my mind I was assuming that just because I'm a
black woman

	that she's assuming that I'm on the welfare system
DELLA:	That you're on welfare . . .
RUTH:	and mind you,
	there are young women my age who, you know
	have benefits from the government, if you will–
	but just
	to look at me because I'm black
DELLA:	Right. Right, right.
RUTH: a	and ask me for it, you know, my Medicaid card, that
	really made me feel
	you know, embarrassed. I
	felt like, well, maybe I should just get off the
	system because
	I'm not, you know, I'm not *using* the system. I'm not a
	welfare mom or welfare parent. It just sort of made
	me feel bad.
DELLA:	So that
	so that when she assumes
	that because you're black
	and you're on Medicaid
	that . . . you are this stereotype of the welfare mom . . .
RUTH:	Yeah, that's what—that's how—that's how I felt, and
	there've been other occasions when I've taken a Medicaid
	card in to the pharmacy, and
	there's been people ahead of me, I mean:
	I've worked in a pharmacy before and I know that
	generally you don't just ask for a Medicaid card, you
	know, you ask for the *insurance*.
DELLA:	Mm-hmm.
RUTH:	And I've noticed that
	with myself and other women that I know
	we're automatically asked, you know, to give our
	Medicaid card or
	you know, we're not asked what insurance company are
	you with, do you have a co-pay card. We're automati-
	cally asked, um, "Do you have your Medicaid card
	with you?"
DELLA:	Mm-hmm. Mm-hmm, mm-hmm.

RUTH: And that . . . you know . . .
         that poses a problem for me. It's like I said, I think
         insurance is insurance, and I don't think there should
         be any
         you know, difference.

At the pharmacy, Medicaid signified a class difference that was all but whited out at the doctor's office. *Seeing* that Ruth was black, the office receptionist produced Ruth as "black" and consequently as welfare dependent: "she automatically assumed / that I was on Medicaid, and there's no /indications on Ifra's record that she was on Medicaid / because this was a new doctor that she was going to . . . in my mind I was assuming that just because I'm a black woman / that she's assuming that I'm on the welfare system." For the receptionist color signified class; whiteness as noncolor or race-lack neutralized class. It left the white woman's social status *an open question*. The white woman was greeted with *not knowing*: "the receptionist asked her / about her insurance status. She was like, 'Who are you insured by?' and she [the woman in line] gave her her Medicaid card. She [the receptionist] / didn't say anything else." Ruth, on the other hand, was met with *knowingness*.[21] The receptionist knew her before she could speak. As Ruth said, "when it came to *me*" the receptionist pointedly asked, " 'do you have your Medicaid card with you today?' / As if / I couldn't have insurance or wouldn't be insured by . . . a company per se." Ruth's dark skin was hypercharged with assumptions about class, sexuality, and dependency, compounded in narratives of the "welfare mom."

Similarly privileging whiteness as noncolor or race-lack, the pharmacist positioned Ruth within discourses of race, gender, and class that, in handing up her Medicaid card, she effectively guaranteed. She closed the gap between skin color and discourse—and paying for prescription drugs became something else altogether: a ritual marking, a consolidation of self and skin color within what Fanon calls a "racial epidermal schema" by which he says: "I am given no chance. I am overdetermined from without. I am the slave not of the 'idea' that others have of me but of my own appearance" (Fanon 1967:112, 116). Accordingly, race is less an idea—internalized, challenged, dismissed—than it is the material effect of embodied social relations. It is produced in rites of "epidermalization," rites so common as to comprise a net of everday transactions (Fanon 1967:11). Organized in "a dialectic of inside/outside" (when blackness is "the constitutive outside of whiteness"), "the discourse of race claims and incorporates the body as its truth-effect" (Pellegrini 1997:103, 92, 102).[22] It makes the body perform its truth. As Fanon argues:

A slow composition of my *self* as a body in the middle of a spatial and temporal world—such seems to be the schema. It does not impose itself on me; it is, rather, a definitive structuring of the self and of the world—definitive because it creates a real dialectic between my body and the world. (111)

Accordingly, at first Ruth felt embarrassed. Then the full force of the pharmacist's assumptions, made palpable in the exchange of her Medicaid card (her hand to his and back again), receiving the drugs, *not* making a co-payment, walking out of the store *raced, classed,* and *ashamed,* began to hit, and she began to feel guilty, so guilty that it seemed the only way she could avoid being class/welfare/welfare abuse-identified was to "get off the system" that abused her. The pharmacist or receptionist's "automatic" request for Medicaid information worked its performative power. It positioned Ruth, and, as she says, other young women like her, in a complex narrative that she could get out of only by getting off the Medicaid /welfare rolls.

And yet Ruth had worked both sides of the counter. She'd been both a pharmacy cashier and customer. Again, her double identity produced a keen sense of contradiction: she knew that her guilt was the effect of an arbitrary element in a ritual exchange, but knowing this didn't make her feel any less guilty. Nor did it enable her to "get off the system" on which she in fact depended for basic medical care for herself and, later, her child. It did inspire her, however, to draw all the contradictions she'd seen and experienced into her "ingenious plan." At the hospital admissions desk she did not hand up her Medicaid card. She refused to let her story "be absorbed by the central story" (Steedman 1986:144). She submitted instead the sign of another self—a card indicating coverage on her mother's company plan—effectively making herself *un/known.*

Rather than getting off the system, Ruth slipped through it and, having slipped through it, said: "I felt more at ease knowing that I had sort of pulled a game off, pulled the wool over their eyes with the insurance because we knew it had lapsed. / I just felt more comfortable knowing that, / and I was treated so nice." Ruth obviously felt better being in a single room, being treated well, but, as she told her story, these common comforts seemed entirely incidental to her greater pleasure in knowing what the hospital didn't know: that her mother's policy had lapsed or was about to lapse, that she had tricked the system (she "had pulled the wool over their eyes"), that she had turned systematic race/class *marking* into *masquing*: she performed the "system" that would perform her. She offered up her card like a mask at a carnival ball. She didn't impersonate someone else so much as she invited misrecognition and misidentification, in effect allowing the hospital to position her favorably.[23]

Ruth pulled the trick off in style. She made the anonymous dispersal of power across a range of hospital practices answer to her wishes and needs. She used the hospital's administration of insurance identities against itself, resisting the technocratic production of difference by what amounted to a mere sleight of hand. As a result she was literally named differently. While her cousin was called into place either by her class status as a staff patient or by her first name (in the proprietary mode reserved for menials or servants), Ruth gained the distance manners preserve. She went on with her story, barely able to contain her winking pleasure:

> RUTH: I don't know how I would have been treated
>   otherwise, but
>   you know, I was greeted "Ms. Stevens," and I noticed,
>   too, with my cousin
>   um . . . who was a staff patient on Medicaid
>   they called her by her first name. Not once did they
>   call her
>   by her last name. They didn't greet her as miss, ma'am,
>   or anything, but I was treated so nicely. I was greeted
>   as Ms. Stevens even though I was a single parent. . .
>   um
>   (*conspiratorial tone*) on Medicaid, but— (*both laugh*) had
>   them think that
>   I had insurance. Um, I was greeted, you know, and
>   they treated me
>   with the utmost respect, I didn't have any problems.
>   And um, I was pleased that I had sort of pulled this
>   trick on them.

Ruth kept her secret—and her self—from a massive information system that purported to know who she was by what insurance she carried. In so doing, she exercised a performative ethic.[24] She made do with what little she had—and what she had were the duplicities she found at the heart of the hospital system. She played the system. She appropriated the hospital's strategic manipulation of insurance information for her own ends. She made a livable space for herself in the place of stiff inequities.[25] By reserving rights to the production of her own identity, she practiced what Michel de Certeau has called a peculiarly popular form of wisdom:

What is there called "wisdom" . . . may be defined as a stratagem . . . and as "trickery." . . . Innumerable ways of playing and foiling the other's game characterize the subtle, stubborn, resistant activity of groups which, since they lack their own space, have to get along in a network of already established forces and representations. People have to make do with what they have. In these combatants' stratagems, there is a certain art of placing one's blows, a pleasure in getting around the rules of a constraining space. We see the tactical and joyful dexterity of the mastery of a technique. . . . Like the skill of a driver in the streets of Rome or Naples, there is a skill that has its connoisseurs and its esthetics exercised in any labyrinth of powers, a skill ceaselessly recreating opacities and ambiguities—spaces of darkness and trickery—in the universe of technocratic transparency, a skill that disappears into them and reappears again, taking no responsibility for the administration of a totality. Even the field of misfortune is refashioned by this combination of manipulation and enjoyment. (DE CERTEAU 1984:18)

Switching tickets at the gate, Ruth created "opacities and ambiguities— spaces of darkness and trickery—in the universe of technocratic transparency." She became oblique, untouchable, finally: unknowable. At the same time she enjoyed herself, even as she enjoyed recounting her secret stratagem to me now. She "created at least a certain play" in the order of things, "a space for maneuvers of unequal forces and for utopian points of reference" (de Certeau 1984:18). She awakened a sense of possibility within the tight frame of hospital administration and, more generally, the corporeal schema of race and class. With that play and possibility came exorbitant pleasure, pleasure "in getting around the rules of a constraining space," a sense of "joyful dexterity of the mastery of a technique," enjoyment even in "the field of misfortune." Ifra's birth was, for Ruth, a profoundly ambivalent experience that climaxed, nonetheless, in powerful pleasure, in heartbreak turned to such joy that "it just felt like my heart was going to jump out of my chest":

RUTH: Well, it was
             exciting, it was scary.
             It was—I was mad, I was happy. You know, it was just—
                I don't know, I had all kinds of, you know emotional
             things to deal with because
             I—I don't know, I went through a lot. I mean I was a

young parent
to be, and um I had chosen to
remove myself
from, you know, my relationship with Ifra's father.
And I was—I felt like I was doing something on my
    own even though my mother was there and, you
    know, she wasn't a very good coach (*laughs*). Mind
    you, 'cause she didn't, she didn't know. She was young
    when she had me, of course, so you know she really
    didn't know what to do. But it was—
I was soo . . .
I don't know.
If I could think of one word
I think that
I would say that I was completely *amazed*
And . . . I was asking my mother, "Well, what does it
    mean when your water breaks?" and she was like,
    "Well I don't know!" because she (*sharp laugh*) was
    the same *age* having
a *child*, and I was like, "Well
what's supposed to happen?"
She's like, "Well, I don't remember."
So it was something—it was *new* to me because I
    didn't have
an experience story from her because she could only say,
    "I don't remember" or
or she would go, "back in those days" they would give
you some drugs or whatever to dope you up so
she didn't know, and I didn't know what to expect
    so I—
I read all of the literature, everything that they gave me
    I read and I don't generally like to
read a lot. And, I don't know why but
I just—I was so amazed with everything dealing with
    the birth. I read books about
being a *parent*, I read books about the
    birthing process.
I mean,
I was so enmeshed in

knowing about having a baby
I read everything,
so I sort of knew what to expect. But I just didn't know,
you know, what everything would *feel* like.
And when I went to the hospital I was like, oh, I know
it's got to be time.
I know it's time.
And they, you know, did a little exam and they
monitored me
and it was like, "Oh, Ms. Stevens, you know it will
probably be another couple of days before you
come back."

DELLA: Oh my goodness.

RUTH: I went to the hospital four times (*Della gasps*), and they
told me this four times before I actually went in to
(*gentle laugh*) give birth to Ifra, and that fourth time I
was like, "I'm not going back home"—I live only
about a minute from the hospital. It's walking distance—I said, "I'm not going back home. I *have* to
stay this time. Please let me stay."
And so that—the fourth time, they let me stay.
     And um
you know I just felt the urge
to *push*. I was like, "Well, OK, I'm going to push now
'cause it feels better when I push!" I was just telling
the doctors what I was going to do, and they were
like, "OK, go ahead," you know, "do whatever feels
natural to you." So, you know here I am. There was
no doctor in the room
and the nurse kept going in and out, I guess because
they didn't think—

DELLA: Now how long had you been there?

RUTH: I had been there only about ten minutes (*Della gasps*).
And um, little did I know—they didn't tell me this at
the time—but
Ifra's head had already come down—
past my cervix and, you know, she was about to be
delivered at home, but I didn't know that. And to
avoid scaring me at the hospital they just sort of told

me to push and do whatever comes natural
because had I known her head was out I probably would
    have panicked and freaked out
So
the natural thing for me to do was *push*, and I didn't
    know how hard to push or you know how—how
    much to push. She just said push and . . .

DELLA: And was your mom there then?

RUTH: She was there
she was standing there beside me, but she, you know she
    didn't know either.

DELLA: Yeah.

RUTH: And she was just saying, "Well I think I see something,"
    but you know, she (*laughing*) didn't know.

DELLA: Oh gosh!

RUTH: And I just pushed and
you know
before I knew it
I had a baby. I thought I had a bowel movement.

DELLA: Yeah.

RUTH: And
they were like, "The baby is here," and I was like
    (*exalting*): "The *baby's* here! Well, where's the baby?"
I was just so excited.
I wanted to see the sac. I wanted to keep the placenta.
    I wanted to
do everything, I was so excited.
But . . . um, they talked me into, you know (*laughing*),
    getting rid of the placenta (*Della laughs*). I wanted to
    take it home and freeze it.
(*laughing*) I don't know what I was thinking about.

DELLA: Make placenta soup, that's—I've heard of that one.

RUTH: Yeah . . . I was just so—I was like I'm going to keep *all*
    the afterbirth, *everything*, but you know they . . .
    (*laughing*) talked to me about that.
But I didn't know I had a ba—you know I didn't know I
    had a baby.

DELLA: Oh my goodness.

RUTH: And then they said well—

or rather my mother said (*small, high voice*): "Well, it's a
   girl." And automatically I said, "Well, let me see
   Ifra."
And they laid her on me.
And you know once I had her it was just—it was a
   feeling,
just . . . I mean
I had experienced heartbreak before, you know, and my
   heart felt so empty, but this was a time when I felt
the most love
you could ever feel and
my heart
it just sort of felt
overwhelmed, and it was just so
so full of joy it just felt like my heart was going to
   jump out of my chest.

For all the possibility Ruth's story evoked, it would be wrong to roman-
ticize her achievement, to consider it anything more than a tactical win in
an ongoing battle that entered another phase when she appealed for welfare benefits, just hours before we talked. In the social services office that
morning she could not so easily divert appearances or slip from one identity place into an identity play space.[26] She needed welfare and was consequently doubly vulnerable—to her own need and to those who administered it. There was far less room to move here. The script into which she
entered, even to the extent that it was less formally applied, was rigid, brittle with suspicion. In the hospital Ruth manipulated the means of identity production that controlled not only the maternity patients but the staff,
doctors, and nurses (who weren't *essentially* nasty or nice but whose performances mirrored their patients' assigned roles) as well. She at once passed
for a privately insured patient and embodied "the ambivalent structure of
all identifications" (Pellegrini 1997:111). In so doing, she created some envi-
able mischief and gained parity. She made the hospital bureaucracy answer
to a performative ethic. If she hadn't, she would have been treated—as
Karen was—like trash. From the moment she entered the social services
office, however, she was assumed to be trash. *Walking in*, she didn't have a
card to play: the play was fixed in a conflict between need and control.

Ifra's father had been murdered for unknown reasons by an unknown
assailant two months earlier. He had taken Ifra to visit with his parents in a

town three hours away. His body was found in a wooded area at the edge of town to which he had apparently driven with his assailant and Ifra. The murderer had, apparently, driven Ifra back to a local parking lot where she was found in her car seat, in the empty car, six, seven hours later. In part because he had made sure that Ifra would be found, the unknown murderer was presumed to be "known" to Ifra's father and, by extension, to Ruth.

Ruth and Ifra's father had agreed, as she said, to be "co-parents." For several months he had been taking care of Ifra during the day while Ruth studied and went to class. On the weekend that he was murdered Ruth was taking final exams, anticipating working full-time after graduation while Ifra's father (Ruth never mentioned his name) cared for their child. When she applied for public assistance she was not only repeatedly grilled by police and media investigators about her ex-boyfriend's death but was at a loss for how she would finish school, work, and take care of Ifra. Ruth had been receiving AFDC for Ifra. Now, because she couldn't work, she had to petition for herself as well. She proceeded reluctantly, laughing with recognition at all the contradictions and ironies that characterized this second visit and yet unable to do anything about them, barely able to sustain her sense of self in the face of relentless interrogation:

RUTH: It made me laugh because I saw how I was treated
            differently because
         when I
         I went the first time
         I had a job—I was employed
         and I just wanted benefits for Ifra. And this time going
            back being unemployed
         um, now, being a single parent because her father was
            murdered and, of course
         the whole—when they asked me
         it almost seems like everybody who asks me about his
            murder they say, "Was it drug related?"
         Everybody. You know, I was like, "Well I don't know I
            wasn't there . . . um, hopefully it wasn't." But, you
            know, just . . . the stereotypes of black males being
            involved in drug transactions.

DELLA: And they asked you this at the Social Services?

RUTH: Yes, they asked me that at Social Services today (*laughs*)!
         I was like, "Well, um
         I can't give you an honest answer

because I—I, "*I don't know*" and the police had concluded
that because they didn't find any drug paraphernalia or
items at the scene so, they just found a dead body. You
know?
um. . . so it was just, you know, going through the
process again,
applying for
Medicaid
AFDC
you know, food stamps. I just felt so—
I don't know. At one point I just didn't even want to go.
I didn't want to deal with it because
even today I was asked a million questions, "Well,
well, why *aren't* you working?" And then I would say,
"Well I don't have child care."
Then they'll reverse it back to me like that was
an excuse
and then I'd say, "Well, you know,
I'm still a student.
I—I'm due to go to summer school." Well then they'd
want to know
all these questions, "Well how are you going to go
to school
and you can't go to work?" It's like (*laughs*), "Well, you
know I—"

DELLA: Was it accusatory like that?
RUTH: Yeah, yeah.
DELLA: Like you're trying to get away with something.
RUTH: Yeah! Almost like I was trying to get over
on the system, and I was like,
"That's another issue.
Maybe with work study
I can work and in the past I've been able to take her
with me." 'Cause I was like I had to defend myself
with every interview question, back and forth, I had
to defend myself. And then the thing with "Well,
how do you pay your bills if you don't have a job?
Where are you getting this money to pay?"—and you
know, it was just
back and forth, back and forth. Now—

I can safely say that before, when I did have a job, you
know, they were a lot
easier to talk to and like, "OK, we understand you have
a job and you have a child that you need help with
because the cost of living is high here." And today I
was just treated
completely
different, and the thing with Medicaid, um . . .

DELLA: Because you're not
employed.

RUTH: Employed
at this *time*,
yeah. And I just—I
had to think about that. I was like hmm, it's different
how you're treated
according to your circumstance.
You know? And um
like for some—

DELLA: And according to your
degree of need. I mean you need them more
now
so
you get treated worse.

RUTH: Yeah, yeah, now more than *ever*. Yeah, 'cause I mean, I
said, well, yes, I needed it during the time frame when
I was
having my baby
and up until the point where I could get on my feet.
OK, that was taken care of and unfortunately we had,
you know, a trauma in our family,
and—I need help *again*! You know?

DELLA: I'd say!

RUTH: And it's just almost like, well, they were pointing a
finger at me. That's what I really felt like: they were
pointing a finger at me
because of my circumstance.

DELLA: If you had said that the murder was drug related then
you would
somehow have been implicated in that

RUTH: Yes.

DELLA: you would

be part of a drug culture or something.

RUTH: Yeah

that's exactly how I felt.

Yeah, that's exactly how I felt because, um

(*clears throat*)

at the time

like I said Ifra's father he was doing well about taking
    care of her and, you know, providing. If I needed
    something I'd just ask him and he would do it

eventually. But

the thing is, with them, is, "Well,

how could

how could he support you

if he wasn't working a full-time job?

Was he using drug money?" It's almost like they
    didn't want to

help me, so to speak. I was like, "Well, I don't know of
    any drug money that he

may have used because he's been here with Ifra

every day keeping her since January." You know?

I was in school then.

I did my little work study or whatever

and I came home and you know he was always there. I
    said, you know, "Had he *time* to

do something illegal I would—I would *know* about it!"

(*Della laughs*)

DELLA: Suddenly

you're d—you are having to defend

someone

first of all who's gone. I mean—

RUTH: Yeah.

That's how I felt, I felt like I'm in defense for him, I'm
    in defense for myself, and Ifra.

I—you know, especially with, like, the

the Social Services, the whole process, because

it's almost like they don't want to help

if they feel you're withholding information or
you're not doing your part, so to speak and even now, I
    mean, I was questioned so heavily today about
him and I was like, well, he's—not here any more. He's
    not the issue right now.
It's my child
and me. She needs day care. I mean, we need some
financial help right now because it's like a, a crunch for
    us. This is something we never expected. We never
    experienced it before, not to this degree
and I almost felt like
I was on the stand
just to get help.
You know, they were like pointing their finger at me,
    "Well had you done it this way it wouldn't have
    turned out this way"—you know.

DELLA: And it was one person who was quizzing you?

RUTH: Yeah, this was one worker at Social Services who was
    quizzing me,
and then
I had to go to child services

DELLA: Was she white or?

RUTH: She was a white lady, yes.
But
I've also experienced that at Social Services with
    black workers.
Now,
the difference between the black workers and the white
    ones is that, um

—and this was a statement made
by one (*laughs*)
worker in particular who was black—she was like (*sassy*):
    "Well,
I have to get out and work every day
and *y'all* can just, you know, get—get benefits from the
    government." She said "y'all," and I was like, well this
    is not—
coming in for services is not something, I'm sure, where

black women just think, "Well, I'm going to live on
welfare." They don't pay you enough!
They don't even give you enough to live off of so why
would you want to make it a career of living off of
the system when you're not even given enough to
live on?
And she was—you know she kept making comments
like, "Y'aaall." And I was saying, Well just because
I'm here
you shouldn't classify me in a group of other people who
may take *advantage* of the system
or who may be, you know
abusing the system as I see it.

DELLA: Do you know—do you know anyone that does that—

RUTH: I don't personally know anybody who ab—you know,
who abuses—I mean, I don't see how you possibly
could, the only . . . You see interviews on TV and you
see things, but I haven't experienced that in real life. I
don't know anyone who—quote unquote—abuses the
system. You don't get enough.
I mean, if you
especially—for instance, in this town if you can live
off of $236 a month
then tell me how (*laughing*) you can abuse the
system—
and it doesn't go up that much with the amount of
children. I think the most you can get is
a little over $600 and that's for like five kids or so. You
can't live off of that especially here. I said, I can barely live off of that living on campus.

DELLA: You can't get groceries for that.

RUTH: You sure can't! (*laughs*)
That's what I try to tell these people . . .
Ifra's milk is
$2.99 a can.

DELLA: Oh yeah. Yeah.

RUTH: You know.
And I said, I have to get enough to last her, and
it's just awful that you would be

accused and labeled because you go for help. I thought
the services were there, you know to help you, not to
accuse you and abuse you

and classify you as, you know

welfare. You know (*laughs*), that's what I feel like, a
WELfare mom.

And I can imagine how, you know, other people might
feel.

I notice even in the grocery store using food stamps and

I—recently was turned on to, they told me about a WIC
[Women, Infants, and Children] program where I
could get Ifra's milk at a reduced cost or whatever.
But I mean, the reactions you get from people

and especially I notice with other black women

who are

cashiers or whatever, they just sort of—I feel like immediately I'm looked down upon

As long as I'm spending cash I'm treated

like a regular customer, and when I'm spending food
stamps or

WIC I'm

looked at funny, I'm

not greeted at all, and

I'm having things snatched from my hands and having
my groceries thrown in bags. That, you know, that
kind of behavior really bothers me a lot.

DELLA: But I mean that's really hostile.

RUTH: It's *very* hostile

and a lot of times I usually speak up. And, you know, at
times, I've even [looked at people working on the
checkout line] and said, you know, "You're probably
spending food stamps when, you know, you're not
working here."

DELLA: Yeah. Yeah.

RUTH: And a lot of times, you know, that's

the case. I can't really say that to everybody.

But it's just, it's—I think it's just awful that you're
treated, you know,

different.

DELLA: Well, especially I've never imagined
the public nature of that, that they can sort of
make you a show of something with people waiting
behind you in line and . . .

RUTH: I know, and that, that, that's *really*
been—
an embarrassing thing for me
so to speak, and
and after I sort of
looked at my situation and said, "Well, if I didn't have to
be . . . in this situation then I wouldn't be. But right
now I'm—I need help and I'm going to go to the
grocery store, I'm going to go to [a large local grocery
store] and spend my food stamps *proud*ly. Because
this is what I have to do to help me and my child at
this time." And until I came to that conclusion I
would go to the grocery store like (*laughs*) at midnight, you know, after hours because they're open
twenty-four hours, but
you know, now I say I don't—I shouldn't have to *hide*
because I know what I stand for
and I know that if it weren't for our family situation . . .

DELLA: What is it—what do you stand for? You . . .

RUTH: Well, I mean
I'm a proud parent.
I'm
proud that
you know, I've . . . gone to [the university]. I'm
proud that
I'll soon have a . . . college degree, and I know that I
won't always be in this situation, that's how I always
look upon it. I say I won't be, you know, needing this
system forever. It's just a temporary thing for me.

Telling me what she doesn't know ("I don't know of any drug money,"
"I / don't know anyone who— / quote unquote—abuses the system"), Ruth
indicates the grounds on which she is presumed to be hiding what she
must know. Avoiding the grocery store at popular hours, Ruth in fact hides

what she does know: "I know what I stand for / and I know that if it weren't for our family situation . . . "—if it weren't for her family situation, she wouldn't be using food stamps, and she would neither be hiding from the glare of public surveillance nor presumed to be hiding the truth.

In the hospital Ruth became herself by becoming *not-not-me* (Turner 1982:120–121). She came into the hospital an unknown, unnamed "me." She would have played a staff patient, someone she wasn't, a *not-me*, had she not bypassed that role for its *other*, the regular obstetric patient with whom she more readily identified or the *not-not-me* the nurses called "Ms. Stevens." She became, in effect, the *other's other*, ironically producing her *real* and, indeed, proper self. The trick proved *true*. In the welfare office she had to fight off being made into someone she wasn't; she had to withdraw from the densely layered performative assumption that she was a fraud, that she was pretending to innocence, and that she was *really*, well, an unfit mother, a drug-dealing slut: any one of the truth effects produced by welfare discourses. And yet to keep from, directly or indirectly, being called a fraud, being *hailed* into the position of a fraud, or charged with performing in the degraded sense of faking and lying, she had to hide— literally, to stay out of sight, to shop at midnight, to keep her government aid a secret. Charged with hiding, she hid, indirectly buttressing the charge that drove her out of the light, out of the regime of the "valued customer," and into the darkness, where the basic need to keep her baby fed nonetheless did not diminish. Usually outspoken, Ruth didn't want to hide. As she said, she "shouldn't have to hide." But, as her interaction with the Social Services officer indicated, not hiding doesn't make for a particularly good defense. To the contrary, it made her an open target.

Reconstructed within official and tabloid discourses of black masculinity, Ifra's father's body became the mute sign of a secret world, a seamy underworld of drug-dealing and gang violence.[27] In the absence of any facts, witnesses, evidence it was the plain clay of a cultural imaginary in which the black male body is a phantasm of dangerous illicit behavior. For the press and police knowing nothing became knowing everything. The *absence of an empirical logic signified a story* in which Ruth was directly implicated, a story wadded with images of wild sexuality and welfare abuse.[28]

Ruth knew too much to comply with the hospital's easy class distinctions. In the Social Services office, however, she knew too little. She could neither confirm nor dispute the interviewer's assumptions about her and Ifra's father. To the very extent that she insisted she knew nothing, she was presumed to be hiding something. She was caught in the irony that she could no more tell the truth of the situation than she could lie about it; as she said, "I can't give you an honest answer / because I—I, "*I don't know*."

The interviewer took her ignorance to be ignorance *of* a knowledge, ignorance of something she did, could, or should know. The interviewer implied that she was either hiding what she knew or was too stupid to know what she should know.

Ifra's father's death remained, for Ruth, outside the discourses that wanted to claim it. The murder, the death, the baby's plight—these were, for her, what Eve Sedgwick has called "pieces of the originary dark" (Sedgwick 1993:25). But, to that extent, they vexed the interviewer's efforts at epistemological control and what seemed her working assumption that there is no "outside" to discourse, that what appears to be "outside" is only hidden away inside, in a secret pocket as yet unplumbed by the appropriate interpretive device. This is the assumption of much scientific discourse and, in a strange alignment with science, the assumption of much classist, racist, and sexist discourse by which the other is not *unknown*, or opaque in her own right, but *unknowing*, or deliberately ignorant.[29]

What I know is that—female, black, poor, single, young, a mother—from the moment Ruth walked into the hospital or the Social Services office she was the subject/object of intensive institutional scrutiny. As Nancy Mairs has observed, if the body is already viewed with suspicion in Western culture (it is the fleshy, irrational thing over which the mind, the "I" that thinks, that *is* because it thinks, is expected to exert control), then the female body is "particularly suspect, since so much of it is in fact hidden, dark, secret, carried out on the inside where, even with the aid of a speculum, one can never perceive all of it in the plain light of day, a graspable whole" (Mairs 1996:85–86). Elusive, in/visible, the female interior must also be illicit, requiring elaborate surveillance and management.

Within white Western culture the black female is doubly suspect: her dark exterior is taken for a sign of her interiority; it is the marked *outside* of an inside receding with every gesture and black *look*.[30] Raced and sexed, Ruth is twice over the interrogated male subject at the center of Fanon's *Black Skin, White Masks*:

> The white man had the anguished feeling that I was escaping from him and that I was taking something with me. He went through my pockets. He thrust probes into the least circumvolution of my brain. Everywhere he found only the obvious. So it was obvious that I had a secret. I was interrogated. (FANON 1967:128)

Because Fanon's white man couldn't find anything but the "obvious," the black man had to be keeping a secret. The white man's projection of the black man's difference is thus doubled in excess: in what cannot be controlled or contained. The white man in effect produces the very excess that escapes him. He produces the black man as an impenetrable other. In so doing, he reveals his own whiteness—his power mania, his sense of being "one" to the "other." What in fact becomes obvious is that the more relentlessly he pursues a secret he'll never find because it is not there, except in his projections of *secrecy*, the more he is provoked by his inside-other, his abject, spectral self othered in the figure of the black man or woman.[31] To the very extent that he construes black as not-white, he becomes thick with the opacity of being not-black. Whiteness is a mask that, in the end, he must suspect he wears. Performance comes home to haunt him.

As James Scott has observed, when dominant groups suspect that they are paricipating in a performance, an elaborate parade/masquerade of power, they will disavow its inauthenticity in part by naturalizing deceit among subordinate groups. They will consolidate their own position by assuming that "those beneath them are deceitful, shamming, and lying by nature" (Scott 1990:3). They clear themselves of any part in the ambivalent play of what Homi Bhabha calls "mimicry"—the installation of power through the "double articulation" of authority and its excesses—by identifying deception with race and class. They secure power through "the representation of a difference that is itself a process of disavowal" (Bhabha 1994:86). Identifying blackness with secrecy, and secrecy as a so-called natural fact read off the black man or woman's skin, the official discourses of white culture disavow the sham entailed in naturalizing *blackness* as such. By sloughing off their own performativity onto what Fanon calls "the fact of blackness," the welfare agent, the doctor's receptionist, the grocery store cashier—each performs *against* the opacity of his or her own performances, such that: I'm right and true, transparent; she or he is lying, faking, hiding.

But as Ruth noted, whether the welfare officers were white or black, they treated her with the same suspicion, suggesting just how closely bound up race and class are in a "public transcript" that colors welfare *black*. Despite the fact that there are currently many more poor whites in the United States than blacks, it is typically the poor black mother who acquires the title "welfare queen"—who, named and contained as such, anchors both whiteness and white/black middle-class privilege.

Performance is the operative condition of power. It is where the "hidden" and official transcripts of public life intersect and erupt into dialectical interchange (Scott 1990). It is moreover where the "edifying deception" that Ruth performs in the hospital—her "ability to flout widely understood boundaries through mesmerization and alchemy, a subversion of common perceptions of the culturally or physically possible through the creative and deceptive manipulation of appearance" (Dyson 1993b)—meets official mimicry, splitting open colonial power, revealing its disavowals as deceptions, not hiding it away at all but multiplying and democratizing it in the performative play of visibility and invisibility.[32]

Ruth was also subject to normative standards meant to contain and delimit maternity. Birth begins with the performance of a secret: with the tantalizing plenitude of the mother "doubled" in pregnancy. The maternal body hides what it knows and yet, in the corporeal signification of pregnancy, reveals its concealment. It performs its secrecy and so threatens masculinity, paternity, and the state with what they don't know/own. Ruth's baby, her postpartum body, both doubled and redoubled in the generations of women and children that surrounded her—all took up *extra space*. Her maternity put *excessive* demands on white middle-class moralities.

In the face of such excesses medical institutions devote massive resources to penetrating maternal/epidermal surfaces—whether by sonography, chorionic sampling, amniocentesis, or cesarean section, all of which make visible what the abdominal wall blocks from view. All get the female body *out of the way* of the fetus it hides.[33] All have the double effect of conveying information about the fetus and effacing the mother in the name of dislodging the fetal secret from its (criminal?) hideout.

All are consistent, moreover, with the narrative interpretive strategy of "*peeling back* stories to reveal better and better ones" (Plummer 1995:170; emphasis mine) and, on a grander scale, with forms of official state violence committed on women in the name of *getting the truth*, exposing, revealing what the female body, by its very nature, is presumed to hide. All depend, as Page duBois has so cogently argued, on thinking about truth as *that which is to be revealed*, as "the secret, as the thing not known, not accessible to consciousness":

> A hidden truth, one that eludes the subject, must be discovered, uncovered, unveiled, and can always be located in the dark, in the irrational, in the unknown, in the other. And that truth will continue to beckon the torturer, the sexual abuser, who will find in the other—slave, woman, revolutionary—silent or not, secret or not, the receding phantasm of a truth that must be hunted down, extracted, torn out in torture. (DUBOIS 1991:147)

Identified with nature itself—by its fertility, its excesses, its protruding belly and breasts, it extrusions in birth and of blood, its open "grotesque" passageways and permeable boundaries, the maternal body comes in for particularly intense scrutiny.[34] It is no wonder that, as Evelyn Fox Keller has made clear, the project of enlightenment science reproduces itself in a "drama" of triumph over maternal nature:

> The ferreting out of nature's secrets, understood as the illumination of a female interior, or the tearing away of nature's veil, may be seen as expressing one of the most unembarrassedly stereotypic impulses of the scientific project. In this interpretation, the task of scientific enlightenment—the illumination of the reality behind appearances—is an inversion of surface and interior, an interchange between visible and invisible, that effectively routs the last vestiges of archaic, subterranean female power. Like the deceptive solidity of Eddington's table, the visible surface dissolves into transparent unreality. Scientific enlightenment is in this sense a drama between visibility and invisibility, between light and dark, between female procreativity and male productivity—a drama in need of constant reenactment at ever-receding recesses of nature's secrets. (KELLER 1990:178–179)

In Keller's view the female body as body, as flesh and form, is the central problematic of the Enlightenment. Spurred on by its apparently "deceptive solidity," enlightenment (rationalist, positivist) science makes its assault on embodiment itself, overtaking maternity in its relentless and, for Keller, ultimately lethal drive toward clarity.

Still, science depends on representation for revelation. It can discern only a representational real—even in the accumulation of data and statistics. It too has to hide, to condense its performativity in "objectivity." To recognize its representational status would mean recognizing how vulnerable it is to manipulation and misrepresentation. You can't trust the language of representation any more, it seems, than you can a woman: stories are slick, slippery, false; anecdote is weak. By this logic narrative, dialogue, and other modes of performative truth making fall away against the rise of "hard" (or "Hard Copy") interrogation, and interrogation (which always already knows what it knows: that there's a secret out there, in there, untold and invisible) becomes indictment. It is a way to catch or catch *out* its (female and/or feminized) subject in the performance of a masquerade[35]—to get her to yield up the truth, to *break* her, to make her perform *its* truth, to incorporate its penetrating power in feeling defensive, lacking, "embarrassed," "on the stand," basically: guilty as charged.

In this light secrecy, even more than any particular secret or bit of information, is the thorn in the side of techno-transparency. The state needs to know Ruth. It covets her self-knowledge; it wants it for its own. The interrogation thus performs the function of making Ruth *known*—not in any sense related to her personal autonomy or even to the (non)story that clearly troubled the Social Services agent—but in the sense of making her intelligible, readable, according to established codes of subject identity. With each accusation (" *'Well had you done it this way it wouldn't have turned out this way'* " " *'Well / I have to get out and work every day / and* y'all *can just, you know, get— get benefits from the government.'* ") the agent presses Ruth into narrative service. She uses the ritual force of the interview process to make Ruth perform the role she is suspected of performing all along, so that, by the end, Ruth says: "You know (*laughs*), that's what I feel like, a *WELfare* mom."

Coded within this "behavioral vortex," Ruth is drawn into betrayal, not of secrets or confidences, but of herself (Roach 1996:213). She is made to identify against her sense of herself as Ifra's protector and standardbearer and against the sense of history, place, and community she invokes every time she refers to the genealogy of single mothers, the generations of "chatty" women ("my grandmother had four girls, and her mother had thirteen children . . . of the thirteen, I want to say that eleven were girls") of which she is, for better and for worse, always a part.

Caught for a moment in this betrayal, Ruth nonetheless stakes her identity on doubleness. The grocery store cashier had her in a corner. There is a line of customers behind her. She's got to complete the store "exit" procedure: she's on display and she's got to pay with food stamps. Readied for ritual humiliation, Ruth speaks up. She doesn't defend herself exactly but dismantles the cashier's discursive authority with a quick "You're probably spending food stamps when, you know, you're not working here." She turns the tables on the cashier's smug confidence in the stability of her own identity position—and leaves the store secure in the same counterdiscursive knowledge with which she entered the hospital: that race, class, and gender distinctions are fundamentally unstable, that they are culturally, contextually produced, and that they shift as quickly as have the circumstances of her life. Each is, as Ruth says, "a temporary thing." Performing at the threshold of identity places—whether handing over an insurance card or food stamps, entering the hospital or exiting the store—Ruth proves their borders weak.[36] Performing at the threshold of knowing itself, at the place where, for her, meaning and identity collapse into need, she shows, to the contrary, how enmeshed the embodied black, female, maternal self is in discursive reproduction.

Outlying Truths

I.

From the moment I arrived at Ellen's house, I knew I shouldn't have been there. No one answered my knock. The door was slightly ajar. I pushed it open and was eventually drawn into the large kitchen where I waited for Ellen while other people criss-crossed the room, the entrance hall, came in and out of the house, casually, with a sense of shared ownership and open passage. Everything seemed at odd angles—the counters, the people, the crossways, all negotiated by glances and half-talk. I cut straight across the as yet unnamed, unspoken community of friends and relations that had attended Ellen's homebirth just ten days earlier and that tended her and her family now. The house was still dank, still raw with the feeling that somewhere at its center a remarkable event had occurred. I was out of place. I'd crossed a threshold I shouldn't have. I didn't know the language, couldn't con it, and hadn't earned it.

＊＊＊＊

The mid-eighties saw a boom in birthing centers, birthing rooms, single-room maternity care, and certified nurse-midwifery as well as swelling costs of medical care and insurance cuts. In order both to improve care and to build consumer pools, hospitals domesticated birthing rooms, featured luxury amenities (jacuzzi showers, candlelight dinners), and incorporated certified nurse-midwives into obstetric practice. Licensed by state nursing boards, CNMs are registered nurses with secondary training in obstetrics. Their specialized nursing status allows them to satisfy demands for female birth assistance, to provide more constant attention than a physician can typically afford, and to offer "hands on" care—ranging from physical support and perineal massage to manual manipulation of the fetus in utero. Because they simultaneously reduce intervention fees, enable and encourage short hospital stays, and sustain many obstetric practices by providing attractive, intensive, standard but relatively inexpensive care, they are also cost efficient. By the late eighties many obstetric groups had expanded to include at least one CNM, often shifting the staff balance dramatically (the obstetric group that Rachel and I shared, for instance, was comprised of two physicians and five certified nurse-midwives).

And yet midwifery remains a hotly contested practice in many regions, to the extent that at least two practices I encountered could no longer tolerate midwife presence on their staff—despite or perhaps because of the number of patients who preferred midwife care. And in 1983, under intensive pressure from the state medical society, North Carolina (a state that at one time boasted the largest number of practicing midwives in the nation) banned lay or "direct entry" midwifery—midwifery trained in long folk traditions or certified by national organizations that do not require nursing degrees but that are legally recognized by forty-three other states. It did not prohibit physicians from attending homebirths, although it left them subject to stiff professional sanctions (including loss of hospital admitting privileges) and untenable liability costs. Nor did it, except by effect, ban homebirthing.[37] The law abolished lay (unlicensed) midwifery and required certified nurse-midwives to practice in medical settings, under the supervision of a physician. The lay and/or certified midwife who attends a homebirth may consequently be charged with "practicing medicine without a license" and be forced to give up a practice that many midwives feel is a calling. Should a homebirth become seriously complicated for either the mother or baby, the midwife may be prosecuted for additional felony violations, including third- to first-degree murder.

In recent years one of three satellite birthing centers in North Carolina closed for lack of obstetric support; one was newly established by a group of certified nurse-midwives in close connection with a major teaching hospital. The new center can accept only strictly routine pregnancies—no multiple births, no malpresentations, no maternal diabetes or high blood pressure. Many of the midwives affiliated with the new center had previously performed homebirths; most hope to substitute the homelike atmosphere of the center for homebirthing, although not a few remain committed to helping women who still want to birth at home. The number of certified nurse-midwives in the state has risen, reflecting pressures for cost efficiency, but remains low, reflecting the strength of medical warrants on prenatal care and birth.

In general, the centralization of hospital birthing has raised the ante on risk—not only are the mother and fetus presumed to be at greater physical risk in the homebirth (despite evidence to the contrary) but midwives who attend homebirths are at risk of criminal prosecution. At the same time, medicalization has spurred a countermovement, an underground circuitry of lay and certified nurse-midwives determined to provide safe homebirths for women who seek them, for whatever reason—religious, ethical, political, economic (homebirths cost about ten to twenty percent of base charges for a hospital birth, at approximately five to six hundred dollars, or less, often depending on ability to pay). North Carolina law secures medical authority by targeting midwives and by shadowing homebirthing mothers with fear of maternal and fetal fatality. Under threat, super-regulated, mothers and midwives have recreated their marginality, creating "centers in peripheries deprived of stable anchorages" that nonetheless depend on secrecy for safety (Feldman 1991:11).[38]

＊＊＊＊

Five years before I spoke with her, Ellen and her husband had traveled over seventy miles to the nearest birthing center to give birth to her first child, Daniel. Ellen was fully dilated and in transition by the time they arrived. Daniel was breech. His heart rate dropped precipitously. It stayed low. Ellen was quickly transported to the hospital across the street where she received an emergency cesarean section. Soon after the birth it became clear that had Daniel come through the birth canal his hips might have been so seriously injured as to require surgery and ongoing therapies. As it was, at five days old Daniel was fitted for a brace to correct for a turn in his hip bone. Ellen was deeply disappointed by the course of events, but she did not experience her C-section, as she said friends had, "like rape." She didn't feel that she'd been medically assaulted or that she had somehow failed in the birth process. She noted that, "Of course, the birth and his brace are collapsed for me." Consequently, in retrospect, "We felt it was real / fortuitous that it didn't . . . "—didn't work out the way she had planned. And yet, "It, yeah, it's like this unfullfi . . . " Her wavering, unfulfilled claims on disappointment were quickly overtaken by a stronger but vaguer, more distanced description of the surgery: "It's *physically* a very odd experience."[39]

Ellen regretted the C-section but never identified with it. It didn't become the text of her body, her self, the deep story of maternity that she knew it had become for other women. As she said:

> I think when you have a C-section because of failure
> to *progress*
> or you're told your pelvis is too small . . .
> there *must* be some feeling of your failure associated
> with that because it's about your body
> and about *you*.
>
> I didn't HAVE any of that.
> It was about the *position* Daniel was in
> and the amount of stress that he could handle—
> 'Cause it's much more stressful to be birthed

for the BABY
in a breech position.
So, it
   it just wasn't
for me
associated with my body.

The extent to which the surgery can be a defining identity procedure is reflected and perpetuated in the platitude to which many obstetricians still hold: "Once a C-section, always a C-section." Cesareans can be glorious. But they can also be part of a panic discourse that produces a sense that, given precedent, birth is an emergency, a C-section is necessary, the body that had "failed" once will fail again, and the birthing mother who fails to recognize any of this is irresponsible.

Advocating for the possibility of a "vaginal birth after cesarean," the acronymous VBAC movement tried to break the discursive hold of the C-section on the birthing woman. Emphasizing the capacity for vaginal birth *after* a cesarean, it builds into identification with VBAC *dis*identification with cesareans. At the same time, it echoes the norm from which it departs. It names the birth and birthing mother (together tagged a VBAC, as in, "She's a VBAC") by deviation from the law of precedence by which one cesarean section will "naturally" follow another.

Ellen had read and heard numerous VBAC stories. She identified herself as a VBAC. But she seemed no more caught within its oppositional framework than in the discourse it opposed. She operated from a relatively unmarked position, feeling neither particularly dependent on hospital technologies because of the C-section nor resolutely independent of them. She was and remained secure in her sense that "birth was a human event, not a medical situation." I asked her whether the C-section had made her more anxious about homebirthing, as the surgical discourse would imply. Ellen quickly and clearly replied, "No, in fact, what the C-section did was make me terrified to go to the hospital."

Ellen continued to operate under the rule of risk, even terror, but the risk was out there, in the hospital, not in her/her body. In effect, the operative anxiety at the heart of cesarean discourses went awry, sending her away from the hospital into a local underground of midwives willing to perform homebirths. Ellen sought out illicit midwife support while she continued to meet regularly with a back-up physician. She had, as she noted, "double prenatal care." She used med-tech she'd previously resisted—sonography, constant fetal monitoring, clear that she "was not gonna attempt to homebirth if the baby was in a breech position." She welcomed the various means of medical support (IV fluids, oxygen tanks, some medications, maternal and fetal heart monitors) the midwives brought with them. In the end, she agreed to what she called complete "surrender": she would accede without question to her midwives' advice to proceed to hospital care, knowing that her primary midwife had faced "a couple of very bad situations where she had recommended being transported to the hospital and the mother and father refused." She had attended births with each of these midwives. She knew that her risk was their risk, that should she similarly refuse she would be endangering not only herself and her baby but the midwives and the entire circuitry of homebirthing they represented. In what amounted to a secret rite of gift exchange, she tied her last line of protection into the midwives' own.

Ellen's first labor had been fast. She had anticipated that her second would be shorter yet and would come well before her due date. She'd been having periodic contractions for five to six weeks before the designated due date—but didn't actually go into labor until fifteen days afterward. Her midwives and the three friends that would attend the birth were literally on call for five weeks, during which time one friend just moved in and stayed with her.

Indebted to their steadfast patience, Ellen made herself the ultimate "coachable" mother:

> there wasn't anything
> that she told me to do
> during the pregnancy or during labor
> that I did not do.
> I just *did* it
> whether I thought it was a good idea or not . . .
>   (*laughing*)!
> And there were certainly times in the labor,
> the things she told me to do
> *did not* seem like a good idea (*laughing*):
> Laying down on my side did *not* seem like a
>   good idea.
> Walking around did *not* seem like a good idea.
> There were a lot of things that I just surrendered to—
> what she saw needed to be done
> and that *worked* . . .

Like the midwife's gentle admonition, one hand laid on top of her belly, fingers pressed "just a small distance" into the vaginal canal, to " 'start to push *here*. I want to feel it right *here*.' " Or the deep massage that finally eased the baby past the coccyx, after almost an hour of having been "stuck" there—as well as catheterization after a uterine cyst ruptured during labor, adding water and pus to the amniotic fluids thick with meconium that already stained the birthing sheets, constant fetal monitoring, administration of oxygen during the last, long forty-five minutes, and aspiration of the exhausted baby even before her bluish body had fully emerged.

Ellen took in every direction. She let things that irritated her in Daniel's birth—someone talking at her, someone telling her what to do —just "wash over me this time." The birth was difficult. A cervical lip initially closed off the birth canal. Ellen had terrible swelling and tearing—and had to face the baby's suddenly slow descent after almost three hours of pushing. But she gave up on the kind of fighting to which she'd felt compelled in the hospital. She gave up even on the kind of "control" many women seek through alternative birthing methods and to which she was accustomed in her everyday professional life. Under the law of secrecy, in the intensities of mutual risk, she contracted herself to mutual regard. She returned trust for trust, care for care, in equal and rising proportions, such that by the end of our conversation I understood why she seemed to be on the verge of tears throughout, why she and the entire house—her mother-in-law passing in and out, her five-year-old son crying for attention from the bottom of the stairs—seemed still to be quaking with the birth. I don't know how else to say it except that Ellen seemed to me to have been devastated by love. As she said:

> I just opened to receiving
> what was there.
> I will never be the same.
> I will *never* be the *same*.
> Because the experience of being loved was so profound
>   that I couldn't deny it. And that's something very
>   difficult for me.
> It's not very hard to love
> but it's very hard to *be* loved.
> So, I don't,
> I don't think
> there's any
> *closing* that door . . .
> again.

Ellen knew and didn't know that this kind of love was possible. She had seen it, tasted it, but never before had she so fully incorporated it. Never before had she been so fully drawn out of the world of (rugged) individual control into vast love. Now she performed its possibility. In the liminal space of the homebirth she *made real*, made true, what the skeptical management of everyday life made "difficult" even to imagine.

Will that door close? Will the threshold on which we seemed to hover remain open to these deep and transforming truths? Will this, the real, the true, the biggest secret of them all, withdraw, imperceptibly, into its usual (commonplace) hiding place?

Ellen's story was framed by what she called "back-to-back" abandonment and devotion. Her hard lessons in love were made harder yet by the fact that the friend we had in common, who had promised to take care of Daniel during the birth, couldn't wait out the pregnancy. Her husband and children had already moved to another state; she finally left to join them just days before Ellen's second child was born, after repeatedly insisting that she would stay. Ellen found a substitute—who, at the last minute, took a job and who, then, "also backed out." What common sense might call the simple, even unavoidable intrusions of daily life seemed to Ellen violations of a tacit, if not exactly secret, contract to *be there*, to be present, to perform loyalty against all the other claims, ordinary and extraordinary, that "everydayness" makes on our lives (Lefebvre 1987:9). "It was really hard for me to understand," she said. For Ellen, a promise is a promise, even as, for Ruth, insurance is insurance. Neither is conditional. "If I had promised somebody to be there to take care of their child during their birth," Ellen said, "I would be there no matter what." Ellen tried to understand her friend's point of view but couldn't—without sacrificing a belief that had now been hardened, by love and pain, into a life principle.

Ellen went into the birth with a strong ethic of care. She came out with a renewed, deepened sense that promises should be kept "no matter what."[40] Faced with the childlike simplicity of this construction, I felt embarrassed for my friend and for invoking her absence by my presence— but also for all of our generally oversophisticated ways, for our jobs and moves and the sense of everyday necessity that nag at the standards for friendship that Ellen's birth held out, held up, and dared me there then, even now, to keep. I didn't know if I could. I don't know now whether I'd want to. Part of me resists the structural asymmetry of life and birth it suggests. Part of me, retreating now, backing off from the doorway I never felt quite right entering, withdraws into that place where her story began, where it's a lot easier to love than to be loved, where being out of control means fighting to regain it. Part of me is already gone. Allied with the friend who first left her, who was not *there* at the critical moment, I carry the scent of her absence, abandonment, and the threat of betrayal she had come to symbolize for Ellen. I am the outsider to be guarded against. I have, at least in part, produced the interiority at whose edges I hover.

And yet I am, as I suspect Ellen will be, forever inside the secrecy she performed. I don't have any privileged information about Ellen's birth or homebirthing. There was nothing of the conspiratorial whisper in our exchange, none of the "Shhh, don't tell anyone else" and "no one is allowed to know this" of what Toni Morrison calls "back-fence" intimacy (Morrison 1993:212). To the contrary, Ellen told me what she wasn't going to—and would never—tell me, by explicitly *marking* the anonymity of "the three midwives" who attended her birth, at least in part by repeatedly referring to them as "the three midwives." She performed the "fragile insulation" that not only protected the midwives from recrimination but that helped her build and sustain this center on the periphery of regular, regulated ways of interacting, being, birthing. She spoke almost unerringly in a plural voice, speaking for the anonymous midwives, neighbors, and friends who assisted her, their numbers expanding, it seemed, with each reference. Telling her story only ten days postpartum, Ellen seemed to double and double herself again in identification with her birth assistants, their colleagues, and other women elsewhere now drawn together in mutual secrecy and accomplishment.

Like Andrea, Ellen didn't particularly need me. Our conversation was easily diverted; it occasionally faltered. I felt part of a second, even secondary, order of exchange. The midwives made up her primary narrative environment (Schrager 1983). It was with them that she was still sharing, comparing, and composing what would become stories of the birth. It was from them that she acquired the string of "birth beads"—a rosarylike string of beads, each one added by a mother who also added her story to a book that is sometimes passed along informally, sometimes lodged at a local women's health clinic—that she held during the birth. The book and beads were, for Ellen, "more than a number of stories." Beyond the information or strategies they conveyed, they "called on the power / of remembering all these women had done this." They were a charm for the "power of remembering" and a sign of collective agency. Holding them, remembering with them, anticipating adding to them, Ellen mobilized memories of women she knew beyond knowing, unknown women with whom she forged something beyond power/knowledge, something more like *pleasure*/knowledge, when power tips over into the pleasures of sensual identification.[41]

Ellen identified her assistants by their sense-presence. She witnessed them now through a shimmering veil of anonymity:

> the primary midwife—
> I was very aware of her visually
> and of what she had to say to me.
> There was one midwife who—her, her *body*, you know,
>   the presence of her *body*—
> I leaned against her body a lot.
> She held me up a lot.
> She rubbed my back a lot.

"The same thing with the friends who were there": Ellen knew them by what they did and how they felt; they remained nameless—not because revealing their names was particularly dangerous but because their felt presence also seemed to supersede the pedestrian business of knowing people by their names. Names individuate. To the contrary, Ellen knew her friends and, reciprocally, her self, in between bodies, in the indistinct space—in the erotic imaginary—of touch and smell:

> I remember
> this one person who I physically didn't see very often
> but there were things like:
> I knew
> at several points she sprayed this *mist* on me that was
>   cool water with some jasmine oil in it . . .
> And I *knew* that was her.
> That was her *touch*.

In this space what mattered was not bodily presence alone (this was not some kind of experiential romanticism) but the telling, sensuous passage between embodied subjects. In the performative relation of body to body, subject to subject—Ellen knew her friends and, in turn, her self. In the process of shifting her bodily alliance from everyday routine to consequently dangerous modes of being, knowing, birthing, she came into an alternative sense of self and knowing and a sense that knowing this way was right and good. A performative relation became a performative ethic that rumbled beneath her insistent "I *knew* that was her," that bubbled up with "That was her *touch*." Telling me what not telling names enabled,

Ellen told a secret she had suspected others knew but that she had never, until now, been close enough to *touch*. Now she felt she knew it irrevocably, that it was imprinted indelibly on, in her body-self. It was this knowledge, coupled with the need to protect the midwives that made it possible, that required whatever tender boundaries she could secure.

Once or twice Ellen had to catch herself. She stammered or paused, almost breaking the code of anonymity, almost telling the secret. But, when she did, she only punctuated the extent to which *not* naming names had become a performance in its own right, suggesting above all the elusive presence—everywhere, nowhere, anywhere—of nurse-midwives willing to sacrifice their lives and licenses to homebirthing. Having entered this liminal domain of *knowing secrecy*, I was consigned to not knowing anything.[42] I didn't have any of the kind of knowledge that would let me pin a name to a face, and a face to a function, and/or a function (domestic midwifery) to the wall. I knew this group of women was out there somewhere. I also knew that I could locate them if I needed to or wanted to—but I didn't want to. I enjoyed the way Ellen's secret expanded with each reference to "the three midwives." I liked the feeling of sharing secrecy with strangers, of being inside looking out at people I couldn't see but whose power, presence, and promise I could, more important, *feel*. I liked not being able to violate the secrecy I was privileged to know and, knowing, to protect, even as it extended to include more people I'd probably never know, except by passing reference or their place on a string of birth beads.

Outside the law, creating a center on the periphery of official domains, Ellen turned the outside *in*, making what she took to be crude legalities and thin loyalties the constitutive outside of the world she now inhabited. Ellen made a virtue of inside/outside dualities. She secured them for her own ends. But from inside the new center she thus (re)created, she turned necessarily stiff dualities into another kind of doubling: she amplified the body politic of homebirthing, projecting from the inside out a community whose reach and power was as vast as it was nameless.

2.

Andrea provided one kind of "horizon" story; Charlotte another. Not because her birth was horrible. It wasn't. It was accidental. It occurred outside the scope of story and surveillance. It was *untold*—and so, it seems, told over and over again, in second- and third-hand versions and in Charlotte's own monologic rush to narrative.

Charlotte began speaking the moment I arrived. I'd made some casual remark about how steep her street was. She immediately claimed my comment for her story. "Right, right," she laughed, "but the problem, for me, that's relevant *here* / is that when the ambulance finally showed up / they couldn't make it in the driveway!" She went into the house; I followed. She came out again; I kept following. "Well, he wasn't a good driver anyway," she explained. "I mean, my neighbor was here to help us, / and she said that he wasn't a very skilled driver / he should have been able to make it in, / and she finally went out and told him to go to *her* driveway, / and then they had to carry me up the hill on the stretcher!" I was suddenly inside a slapstick comedy that came at me in 3D, surroundsound.

Charlotte had been told over and over again to expect the "eternal labor": "Everyone had told us, / first time births take forever"; "prepare yourself for the eternal labor of thirty-six hours or worse"; "the midwives had said: / we're gonna have to fight you to stay home." She, like Ellen, had poured over the birth beads book. She and her husband absorbed the stories they heard, writing themselves into the narrative framework of the *eternal* labor that seemed to swallow them all up. They were ready, above all, to stay home until the appointed moment. They'd stocked up on crossword puzzles, borrowed videos, and even bought a game of checkers:

CHARLOTTE:
> . . . well,
> it was funny, with the checkers,
> that, um, neither of us really knows how to play,
>> and (*laughter*)
> we thought, well, we'll have

CHARLOTTE AND DELLA:
> time to learn![43]

Even as they'd bought a game they couldn't play, they'd become *other to themselves*, even people they weren't: the perfect characters in a story about to happen—that never did.

Charlotte woke up feeling achy. She'd had some bloody show. She went to work, anyway, and on to her prenatal appointment at noon. In the middle of her exam her cervix dilated from one to three centimeters, which the midwife noted was "unusual" but generally dismissed, observing that "a lot of women run around / three centimeters dilated / for weeks, and it doesn't mean anything." Charlotte went on an errand and walked the mile from the parking lot back to her office before she started feeling more cramps, "like before a menstrual period sort of thing," which, she said:

> I hadn't felt in months, obviously,
> and I thought,
> well, that's interesting, but
> I really didn't feel very uncomfortable,
> so I thought, ehh?

She stayed at work until after six and then got ready for a rare dinner out (Italian food being reputed to induce labor). She was starting to feel "kinda uncomfortable":

> but it was, so . . . intermittent,
> it was like, every twenty minutes, or so
> and I really didn't pay much attention,
> and then I guess,
> it was about seven or so, . . .
> ya know, I just started having second thoughts about
>   going out to dinner but, I mean,
> that's . . . still very mild at that point—
> do you call that labor?
> Naww.

By the "eternal labor" yardstick, this wasn't labor; it "was no big deal." Charlotte wasn't in labor because she wasn't *in* the thirty-six hours/five minutes apart labor that left her only two options: to be a wimp or to wait out early labor for the *real* thing, for a reality she knew only in/as story. At 8:30 (after they'd abandoned plans for dinner), Charlotte finally felt uncomfortable enough to lie down on the couch, castigating herself the whole time for failing against the narrative standard she'd set: "I said, oh Charlotte, this is so early in labor, you *wimp,* / you don't wanna lie down." And minutes later, when back-to-back contractions made it impossible to time their frequency and duration, she complained of what she presumed was her special incompetency: "How do people *time* these things? I felt really stupid, everyone *times* their contractions, it's a very basic thing to do. / . . . am I incompetent—or what's going on here?"

Charlotte teetered on the edge of a story she'd learned too well, the story in which she'd so carefully plotted her birth, herself, her family, her embodied social identity. When, within minutes, the contractions were rolling on top of each other, everything was up for grabs. She didn't know what was going on: "I didn't know how to interpret it really." The narrative failed her now, even as she finally gave in to what she later called a "classic" transition period: "Wimp or not, I've gotta go lie down for real."

Noting now that "nobody tells you it can happen that quickly" (another secret), she then rallied for whatever anyone had told her—what the midwives had said, what "people say":

> I needed to go to the bathroom (I had developed some
>   diarrhea earlier),
> and I remember the midwife and also our Lamaze coach
>   saying,
> empty your bladder as often as you can,
> 'cause, you have to make plenty of room for the baby to
>   come out and stuff,
> and you'll be more comfortable,
> so I thought, all right, so I'll drag myself to
>   the bathroom,
> and,
> so I got there, and
>
> all of a sudden,
> I felt like my whole body just kinda balled up,
> like, pulled itself together.
> And it wasn't until that moment that I realized how far
>   along I really was.
> And, it was . . . sort of a shock.
> and there's nothing I could have done to stop it
>   people say,
> oh yeah, they told me not to push—
> there's no way I could have *not* pushed!
> And, in the next moment,
> I felt the head coming down.

DELLA: Oh my God!

CHARLOTTE:

> And I said, *THOMAS* (*Della laughs*)!
> But, but at that point when I had gone into the
>   pushing stage

it was the first point that I had any letup from
the pain,
it was all of a sudden an interval with no pain.
It was wonderful,

and then, he tried to call the clinic,
and they had a tape recording to tell you who's
     on call,
and then you call the midwife who is.
Only, at that point he was more excited,
and he couldn't catch the number that they were saying
     on the tape recording (he's Danish, and English is
     only his second language)
so he called the neighbor who had coincidentally just
     gotten off the phone herself,
and said, Marie, could you come down!
She said later that the tone in his voice, the difference
     between a quarter after nine and that phone call

DELLA: Oh boy,

CHARLOTTE:

was really dramatic,
and so she came running down and her daughter
     said too,
she said, I didn't know what was going on
but you never run in the house mom,
you never run and you ran out the door.
And, so she was kinda worried,
and so Marie came down and she made the phone call
     to the midwife,
and meanwhile, Thomas came dashing into the
     bathroom,
and it just felt so good to stand up,
I thought that was the reason the pain had changed,
and he said, no Charlotte, you better get into bed.
And at first he didn't really believe me that the head was
     that far along,
and it kind of went,
that fast.

DELLA: Immediately, you knew it was the head and what was
     happening?

CHARLOTTE:

> Yeah.
> It's like having a huge bowel movement, only,
> I mean it's like one you never had before,
> and you say, oh, this must be what's going on,
> and, um, so he kinda felt in there and said,
> oh yeah, the head is coming.
> And so he sort of steered me back into the bed,
> and Marie brought a bunch of towels that they
>   stuffed under me,
> and um,
> well, he was born at twenty after 10:00.

But Charlotte's son was twice-born, once at home, accidentally, and then again at the hospital, where all the rituals of birth were performed after the fact, like a church wedding after an elopement—doubling the birth as a " 'double medical emergency' " in which both the mother and baby are at risk.[44] For the hospital, the birth was doubly urgent; for Charlotte, doubling up home and hospital had the perverse satirical effect of funhouse mirroring. Here's when the real comedy began. The birth Charlotte now describes as something out of Oz—"I felt like, / you know, in the *Wizard of Oz*, when Dorothy's house just goes up and she looks out the window / and everything's flying by / and she sees these little bits of things clearly— / that's what I felt like / was Dorothy / just—whooooop! (*tornado sound*)"—had just settled down into a kind of grainy, gray-scale peacefulness when the Keystone Cops arrived.

The story didn't happen. To the extent that it did, "it all happened backwards." The baby was born before normal birth routines could be implemented. In effect, the story was over before it began. When the rites of medical practice were performed, they proved hopelessly late, unnecessary, out of step, and off-kilter. Like a movie running in fast-reverse, what might have seemed normal and natural suddenly looked silly. All the attempts to make up for the fact that the birth had slipped even the midwives' cautiously alternative routine looked *backward*—clownish, clumsy, stupid even, not in the usual sense of barbaric—to the contrary, supersophisticated, overregulated, and hyperreal.

The backward-run on birth began with trying to get the midwife on call on the phone. I could barely keep up with Charlotte's account of the missing midwife:

the midwife
that was on the tape-recording was actually not on
    call—it was an error
and so (*laughs*) Marie [their neighbor] got through to
    that midwife who,
well, she wasn't even *home*—
Her housemate told Marie: "no, it's not Sharon [who
    was on call], it's Jules—
and Jules is in the hospital: have her paged."
So, poor Marie calls the hospital and has Jules paged,
and then toward the end of the birth process,
the midwife *was* on the phone,
and she said, "Check his color and do this and that" but
    he was already born, basically.

Then there was the sound of the ambulance wheels spinning in their driveway. The ambulance drivers couldn't handle the gravel or the cut of the hill; the neighbor, Marie, directed them to her house at the top. The paramedics finally managed to get Charlotte on a stretcher and carried her up the hill (as Charlotte said, generously, "They were young and strong-looking and all, but they seemed to have a lot of problems with getting me on the stretcher, / and then they had *a lot* of trouble getting me up this hill"). Once they retrieved the baby that they'd left back at the house (where he'd reportedly said his first "hiii!"), they sped off to the wrong hospital. Thomas had driven to the right hospital where he was greeted by the waiting midwives: "'Oh, / you're the father who delivered the baby at home!' / and he says, 'Yeah,' / and they say, 'Well, where's the mother and the baby?' / and he said, 'I don't know!'" They had in fact ignored Charlotte's instructions and taken her to a hospital within closer range, all the while trying repeatedly, unsuccessfully, to hook her up to an IV drip, insisting, against her claims to the contrary, that she was "woozy." When they wheeled her into the emergency room (Thomas had yet to catch up), Charlotte imagined herself in the ultimate stock comedy routine:

So they wheeled me into the emergency room and
in that reception area there's that counter
and there was a woman standing behind it,
and the driver didn't say anything,

> and the woman kinda looked, and said, "Well, what's
>   the primary diagnosis here?"
> It could have been a gunshot wound for all
>   they knew,
> and they still didn't say anything, so I lifted my head
>   and said, "Birth!" (*laughter*)
> I wish someone had a video camera; it would have been
>   a great scene in a movie!

Routine now took on a new meaning. Out of joint with reality (running up a down escalator), routine became a parody of itself, sometimes funnier than at other times but in general following the comic rule Charlotte had discovered inductively—"It was funny because we actually anticipated the opposite."

The birth had run ahead of performative routine, making a gentle mockery of the phone messaging system, the ambulance, the hospital procedures—all the modern conveniences through which birth is usually monitored and conveyed. The doctors hastened to recuperate Charlotte to their routines, to restore the priority of their methods and to make the birth fit the normative pressure of the story Charlotte had not only anticipated but welcomed. But in that story Charlotte is the subject and not the agent of a birth she had now already *given*. Her agency couldn't be unmade into dependency on the machinery of medical practice. In the end, though, hoping to get "this show on the road," she pretended to complacency. She let the doctors proceed with their compensatory routines:

> At that point I was having contractions again for the
>   afterbirth thing
> and I said, "Let's get this show on the road."
> It seemed like there were swarms of people around—
> lots of med students and residents and all sorts
>   of people.
> Finally they got me in this other room and had me get
>   on this bed that I thought I was always slipping off of
> and all these people were pushing on my stomach
> and *nobody* said anything—I had always wished that
>   they had communicated
> that they had said, We're gonna deliver the
>   placenta now,
> or something

They just sort of started, pulling on it,
and I said, "Do you want me to sort of push or
    something?"
and he said, "If you want to" (*Charlotte and Della
    laugh lightly*).
And I guess at that point it slipped into the vagina
anyway so it was no big deal,
but still,
when I did push it just plopped right out.
It just made things easier,
And they said, "Oh we're gonna give you a shot now," at
    least they warned me about that,
and I said, "A shot of what?"
and they said, "Pitocin,"
and I knew what Pitocin was for and I said, "Why, am I
    bleeding heavily?" And he said, "No."
I said, "Is the uterus not contracting right?"
And he said, "No, hard as a rock."
And I said, "What's the point then?"
And he said, "Oh, well, ya know, it could soften up in a
    half hour or so,"
and I said, "Why don't we wait a half hour or so and
    then you can give me the shot after that."
And I guess they're not used to having people talk back
    to them or ask questions or something,
And he said, "Well it's just routine! Everybody gets a
    shot of Pitocin after birth."
And I knew that wasn't true—
I know other people who've delivered there who said
    they didn't have a shot afterwards.
And the midwife had said, if you have a very fast
    delivery that they sometimes do, if you're having
    problems because the uterus sometimes doesn't
    contract correctly,
but it was,
so I just said, I'm not gonna fight it
and got the shot,
and it wasn't till then that I felt really nauseous and sort
    of irritable, from the shot, I guess.

The wheels kept churning. The resident on duty insisted on blood studies because Charlotte's blood type is Rh negative, indicating possible Rh incompatibility with the baby's father. Charlotte insisted in turn that she already had the same studies done at the same hospital just months earlier and that her husband was also Rh negative, so the studies were moot. The resident returned, "'It's routine, we have to do this'"—and they did. As Charlotte noted, "It basically came down to that they didn't think it was possible / for a woman to be *that* sure who the father / really was."

Unseen, unwitnessed, outside the order of things, Charlotte's accidental homebirth propelled her into discourse. She and Thomas sent complete accounts of their son's birth (double texts: in English and Danish, for their European relatives) with his birth announcement. Charlotte told her story to me—a complete stranger, except for an acquaintance in common and the fact that I (as she had carefully determined) worked for the university—in effusive detail, drawing me into what seemed an elaborate form of narrative surrogacy. This was her birth four times over. It was at least the fourth composition of, first, the birth that seemed to lack a representational reality because no one saw it and no story foretold it, second, the birth routine running on empty, and three, the elaborate, detailed accounts she and Thomas wrote and distributed with their birth announcements. I attended her birth, witnessing it now in the complicities of narrative performance, seeing what she saw, heard, thought, and felt, replayed by understudies, understories, replacements for the eternal labor story Charlotte had been so ready to perform. The eternal labor story was legitimate theater. Without an audience, without a proper script, Charlotte's birth verged on being illicit, a phony, a fake, nothing, "pfffft!" She needed the certification conferred by witness. She also needed and wanted to make up for feeling "gypped," for having been cheated out of being able to tell the story she'd planned to tell and still wanted, it seemed, to be able to tell:

> It feels, it's funny that when other women talk about
> their labors, or their birth experience,
> or whatever,
> It's always, well
> ya know, "the contractions started,
> and we were timing this and that, and,
> then the labor took this many hours"—
> And

And I, I feel almost like I missed out,
because, after all this preparing,
and the breathing exercises,
and the relaxation [exercises], and everything else,
I feel like I don't have that experience to share with
    other women,
because it just went, pfffft!
ya know: all of a sudden, there it was.

The "experience" Charlotte wanted to be able to share with other women was in fact a certain kind of story: a story that followed clock time and the rules of narrative sequence. Her birth occurred in a flash, in another time, outside time. It was not prediscursive as much as it was beyond both narrative and scientific control. It was an accident produced, to some extent, by the very narrative it exceeded. The eternal labor story sets up a double-sided birth script (this is labor, that isn't; this is the right, good, and strong thing to do, that isn't). It writes birth and the birthing mother into a predictable and narrowly moralistic course of action. In so doing, it sets up an outside to the story—not the bad side, the wimp side, but the shadowy, secret border space of neither side, "neither/nor," where deliberation, predictability, and control get stood up by accident: by the unpredictable play of body discourses and by the sudden need to improvise, to perform without a script.

Accident in turn makes *the* story—whether told by doctors, midwives, expectant mothers, husband-coaches intent on doing their jobs well by keeping their wives home—only *one* story among many, diminishing the authority it had assumed in Charlotte and Thomas's lives, as both an interpretive device and as a mechanism of control within, again, a trickster world, a world ready to split and slip narrative, a world that made birth by the clock ("It's always, well / ya know, 'the contractions started, / and we were timing this and that, and, / then the labor took this many hours' ") answer to renegade body talk. Charlotte's baby/body/new maternity tricked her out of her coveted role in *the* narrative into a ravishing replay of images ("I felt like my whole body just kinda balled up," "It's like having a huge bowel movement, only, / it's like one you never had before"), taglines and slogans ("'Well, what's the primary diagnosis here?'" "'It's just routine!'"), other stories ("I know other people who've delivered there who said they didn't have a shot afterwards"), inside stories ("Her housemate told Marie: 'no, it's not Sharon [who was on call], it's Jules— . . .' "), and nonstories ("*nobody* said anything").

Inside the eternal labor story Charlotte also saw herself as she suspected others saw her, performing herself as other to herself, subjecting herself to an internalized surveillant gaze: "I said, oh Charlotte, this is so early in labor, you *wimp*, / you don't wanna lie down." Out from under the eye / "I" of this narrative, however, she took countercontrol of the spectacle. She reimagined herself through *The Wizard of Oz*, trained her dialogue on the doctor's stubborn refusal to ante up: "And they said . . . and I said . . . and they said . . . and I said . . . and he said . . . and I said . . . and he said . . . and I said . . . and he said, 'Well it's just routine!' " all the while wielding an imaginary video camera, reframing emergency room practice as performative antics, declaring: "it would have been a great scene in a movie!"

Taking her authority from the agency she'd performed in birth and her materials from the "elsewhere" her birth embodied—from the in-between places and imaginary spaces left to the margins of the eternal labor story, Charlotte crossed through whatever lack or deprivation she felt. She wrote into the space of her "missing" story, jealously guarding her right to a story and fervently scoring the performance she'd already given. Charlotte lacked conventional scripts and official witness. Lack gave her license—to recreate her unseen world with wild-eyed, yearning, demanding exuberance. Performing out of this particular nothing, she bypassed verification procedures, factual analysis, and validity measures. As hard as the hospital staff tried to reclaim Charlotte, her story—in form and substance—left scientific control in its dust. A story of stories, it was a quintessential performance of a kind of history that is knowable, legible only as story, in the exchange of telling bodies, performing birth: a kind of history that disappears into its representations and that, in performance, disappears into reckoning and remembering and even refusing to reproduce—into making history all over again.[45]

The hospital staff also performed in the place of a lack. A double lack. Charlotte's birth was, first of all, presurveillant, prepanoptic, unseen/invisible to official hospital discourses. As such, it proved those discourses lacking—lacking sense and lacking a subject. The paramedics practiced on a "woozy" woman, the staff performed a second round of blood studies on a woman who, apparently because she was a woman, couldn't be sure who was the father of her child, the doctors tried to administer Pitocin to a woman who should have been dead quiet on a gurney. Charlotte was none of these. And the harder the hospital staff tried to recuperate her to their discourses, the more resilient her *secret story* became: the more it revealed

their secret—in this case, not the crude, even brutal administration of subjectivity Ruth found but the projection of the simplest stereotypes onto an
absent subject, a postpartum body, a maternal body as screen for their own
compulsive imaginings. Charlotte concealed nothing (even answering for
the paramedics who seemed so confounded by the receptionist's routine
question, "'What's the primary diagnosis here?' 'Birth!'") and revealed
everything. Because Charlotte had already given birth, because the show
was in fact over before the curtains opened, what was *shown* (and shown
up) was the hospital's script for birthing mothers. The paramedics and
doctors kept trying to penetrate Charlotte's *secret* world with their instruments, to make her birth legible (and legitimate) by their standards—but
in the end the joke was on them. Their secret was out: their procedures
were, at least in this instance, unnecessary, superfluous. Charlotte's *secret*
was the hospital's understory, the backside and outside of the story they
wanted to tell or had to tell. But, lacking a proper subject, their story made
no sense. It even seemed weary with nonsense: a farce whose edge had
been worn dull.

Did all this make Charlotte prefer homebirth? No: "I mean, enough
births have complications that I would never have purposely had the
baby at home, / I, I would not be comfortable planning that because if
there *were* a complication / and something happened to the baby I would
just feel so guilty about it, I would feel awful. . . . No, I don't really think
it has changed my attitude." In the end Charlotte's homebirth was an
accident, not (as it was for Ellen) an ethic. It had the fortuitous effect of
revealing the hospital's stale routines for what they were—but didn't lead
Charlotte to dismiss those routines or in any way mitigate her desire to
be within their protective reach. I suspect that Charlotte will remain, as
she called herself in our conversation, a "troublemaker"—and that whatever trouble she makes for the hospital the next time around will be
informed by the force accident exerted this time. But the accident
acquired that force by accidental means; it was powerful precisely because
it was unplanned. The deliberate speed with which Charlotte was rushed
to the hospital, drugged, and tested seemed ridiculous next to her homebirth, which was not deliberate, which was beyond all purpose: it was
simple, spontaneous, powerful, charged with the vitality of adaptive
human resources, suggesting that where things go wrong they can go
wonderfully right—but, to that very extent, they can also just as easily go
wrong.[46]

Last lines

Down the mail chute letters sail,
coins cross palms for bread—
the earth opens.
—Connie Conant, "Every Purpose Under Heaven"

The commodification of disclosure in what I have called a tabloid culture makes it difficult now to say anything without saying everything, without being immediately assimilated to established codes of understanding.[47] Within the prerogative of these codes anything you say, it seems, can and will be held against you. You will be made legible, clear, within an operational grammar that surely knows "you" better than you know yourself.

This is why, in the end, Carolyn Steedman makes a gesture at withdrawing her story from public view, at returning it to the darkness, to the margins, from which it came. This is why, moreover, Ruth struggled so hard to *manage* the few identity resources that remained to her. This is why, in the end, it seems we have to reacquaint ourselves with the strange pleasures and practice of silence, with the power of speaking silence—not breaking silence or testing taboos or even speaking the unspeakable, saying what no one else will or can say. Silence isn't the problem as much as is *silencing* or the disciplinary exclusion of certain bodies, selves, and stories from the matrices of approved speech, truth, and value. Sustaining the performativity of the secret, as Ruth, Charlotte, and Ellen variously do, is one way of at once marking that exclusion and taking advantage of the duplicities from which it takes its form. Speaking silence, or letting silence speak its own depths—in image, act shadow, or sensation; in furtive and fantastic histories (crossing and diverging), is another.[48]

Despite the illusion of talk show dramas, the world is not entirely knowable.[49] Mysteries pull at the edges of *knowing* discourse, pulling it apart (Margaret will never know whether she did the "right" thing), pulling it down (Rachel and Joe domesticated the miracle of their repro-tech birth by circling it with stories of the paranormal, supernatural, and supernormal), and pulling it up by the roots (Karen un/named the world, Ellen turned its crude legalisms inside out).[50] The most stubborn mysteries (why Deborah suffered a fifth miscarriage, how and why Ifra's father died) seem to invite the most severe administration of appropriate (or understandable and manageable) identities: Deborah's doctor refers her to a counselor for "excessive" grief, the social worker drafts Ruth into the stereotypical role of the "welfare queen." At the outside edge of even these mysteries, however, is the unstoried mystery of where life meets death and of how death trespasses on the sterile grounds of the hospital or, worse yet, intervenes in the life well lived, the life performed against the threat of death, according to the norms and protocols of the good life, the good birth.

Death won't keep out, stay away. It insinuates itself into the place of life, refusing even the most sophisticated means of exclusion. The inscrutable doubling of life in death and death in life is surely the ultimate duplicity in a trickster world. Death, stillbirth, miscarriage—these are the axes on which the birth story spins.[51] They are the silences (unbroken, unbreakable, but not unspeakable) that speak through all these stories—in rolling waves of fear and desire,[52] in slips, stammers, tricks, evasions, and secrecies, in prebeginnings and afterends—in "pieces of the originary dark" and riotous belly laughter, in excess(ive) speech, bursts of "meaning under a veil of words," and scraps, fragments, images of what's not there now but once was (*a baby, a birth, a scent, a promise*), in unmapped narrative routes, the ragged genealogies that keep the last secret: that there is no single origin to identity, stories, or history, that each begins in (creative) contradiction, dissension, and dispersal, "fabricated in a piecemeal fashion from alien forms,"[53] and in the endless questions of purpose, power, and pleasure to which these stories yield:

> *How can women keep the "symbolic capital" of the secret for purposes not only of refuge and protection but, to the contrary, for the expansion of epistemological territories and the subversion of power/knowledge by something like pleasure/knowledge?[54]*

> *How can stories that originate in contradiction, pain, and absence be used against totalizing order and the rampant illusion that everything that is not already known is or should be knowable? What might it mean to speak not only or necessarily truth but silence to power?*

> *Who has the right, the luxury, to remember—or, perhaps more to the point, to forget?[55] to keep herself to herself, to refuse the light: to return her stories to the darkness out of which they came or to perform beyond reproduction, into the strange pleasures of a performative maternity?*

> *When is silence—the deep silence of the open earth, the singular quiet of repose, the beyond-words of exaltation, or the (secret) silences that raced, classed, sexed visibility keep—the story that needs to be told?*

> *When does visibility break circuitries of power? When and how does visibility trick us into keeping its secrets? When is the power of visibility ours and not ours at all?*

How can performed secrecies at once mark and claim silencing for their own ends? How can they challenge the discourses of maternity, technology, medicine, and science that converge on birth rites, by, for instance, diverting an anatomical or salacious gaze (as Lila does), by drawing new borderlines (as Ellen does), by making absence palpably present (as Rachel does), by un/saying ritual discourses (as Karen does), or by hiding in the open (as Ruth does)?

These stories are born in risk. Not so much in the physical dangers of birth but in *narrative* risk, in the process of subjecting *knowing* to the perils of *not knowing* or *unknowing*, even undiscovering the truths and facts that science covets, in the exigencies and im/mediacies of re-membering birth. Every time a woman tells a birth story she puts her body *on the line*, in the secret divide between some of our most carefully guarded doubles: nature/culture, life/death, gender/sex, public/private, inside/outside, in/visibility, in/difference, birth/story, story/silence, exquisite/dangerous silence . . . silence and the tender, reckless, unbearable sounds of pleasure/pain.[56] In between, on the last lines of defense: birth/stories echo with silences that remain, still, to be heard.

Dear Nat and Isabel:

You are everywhere in this book. In its start, in the interviews, in every revision, in its reason for being. In the power, play, transgressions, and recuperations it recounts. In many ways you have made this book. It is yours. Even in drawing me toward this last performance, this final reflection in the form of a letter you won't read for many years, this performance of a possible future, you have kept me deep within the folds of telling stories that have no end, writing a book that has no end, except this provisional gesture at telling again, and retelling, and, in the process, untelling—old stories, newer stories, the story I tell here with the kind of certainty that comes only with thinking for the moment that this moment will not yield to another, that you will not tell me a different story and make my stories of you figments of time and place. And yet this letter is meant to honor that very possibility. No, to perform it: to call that future into the present, as if we were together *then* as we are *now*—and the roughhewn, everyday *now*, so loaded down with other stories, other performances, is perfected in an impossibly open play of identity making. You are making me now, as I write this, calling me as I have suggested earlier in the book, to what I would call a performative maternity: a sense of myself as a mother who no more "owns" stories of your birth, your selves than I do you, who, in telling, is told, over and over again, what I may become and, in that telling, becomes.

I have tried to be a good mother. I have tried not to be a "good mother." As I have indicated variously throughout this book, I have resisted, refused even (stubbornly, you will no doubt add) narratives of the good mother: narratives that wind their way into the smallest gestures of everyday life, holding the mother to impossible standards of self-sacrifice, dooming her—in the least sensual pleasure, in the least regard for her self—to failure, shame, and embarrassment. I have tried to show in this book (beyond the eighties platitude "What's good for the mother is good for the child") that in making ourselves we make each other and make of the everyday world an opportunity for other kinds of self-becoming.

But in so doing I have often felt the sting of being a "bad mother." Over dinner at a restaurant recently your dad quoted someone saying that his wife hadn't been a good mother to her troubled kids; "'She was always writing.'" I shivered and stalled. I kept saying to him, across the table, That was an awful thing to say. How could he say that? I still think it's awful. But maybe partly because I worry that it's true. While I have been writing this book, because of you, with you, by you, you have often been in extended hours at school or I have been too distracted to listen well, too impatient with myself to be patient with you, keeping my responsiveness in obsessive reserve, for this.

Work doesn't seem to be quite so bad anymore in the "big" stories of what makes a good mother. Writing is the worst. It doesn't quite qualify as work. It can be done at home, in stolen moments. It entails, apparently, the secret satisfaction of expressive desires for which both Karen and Andrea, for instance, longed. It requires sometimes ruthless isolation from children, men, other women (I have never learned to write in the patches of nap or play to which other women and men seem to adapt). It provides few, if any, usable provisions for the family. It represents the lure of attention and authority that women speaking (that the women who spoke with me) don't always or even usually get. The woman who writes is the opposite of the good mother: she holds back on her (pro)creativity for the publication of images and ideas. You are there in those but not here now, as I write, except in the way my thoughts of you ripple through my writing self, driving me to listen harder to other people's stories and to bring them, with yours/ours, into the folds of public knowledge. Because of you I have listened to others. I have performed in writing, sometimes instead of in talking, touching, and staging, our narrative rites.

You might have preferred another kind of mothering. I can only take heart, Nat, in how ferociously you forgive ("Of course, I'm yelling," I yelled one late night when you WOULDN'T go to sleep and I wanted to work, "I'm only human!" "Of course, you're human," you yelled back, tears and sweat smeared across your golden face, "you're my mother, aren't you?"); Isabel, in your persistence to get what you want or need, in your own stubborn desire to be alone sometimes, in your beautiful "made up" poems and songs. And now, as I approach this end, I have to wonder whether had I not-written would I have not-mothered. I want to believe that whatever deferral I performed in the end entailed *refusing the refusal* Steedman performs, even as I meet you here, now, in the afterwords of this book.

I am closing this book then with a hope and a promise. The hope is that in writing this book I have in fact become a better mother—more attuned to "being told" and, in being told and telling again, conveying something of the power—awful, playful, great—of telling, challenging, refusing, even making up birth stories. The promise is an easy but not a simple one: that I will always listen to your stories, thrill to our stories, and become over and over again, unpredictably, neither a good mother nor a bad one but yours.

With all my love.
5/17/97

INTRODUCTION

1. Regarding contemporary U.S. birthing practices as ritual performance, see, among others, Davis-Floyd 1992; Jordan 1993; Leavitt 1986; Michaelson 1988; and Rothman 1991. Birth storytelling as a normative rather than a primarily descriptive practice has been partially addressed by Carpenter 1985; Martin 1987; Peterson 1987; Ruddick 1989; and Schely-Newman 1995.

2. A common literary and media equivalent involves positioning miscarriage as plot relief, as a way of eliminating a pregnancy that has served its plot function by complicating a romance or forcing moral reflection and yet that would overdetermine subsequent events should it remain. For example, in Maeve Binchy's popular *Circle of Friends*, a lead character's miscarriage is announced at the end of one chapter and the next chapter begins several months later, leaving a gap large enough to say: "Life goes on," as if miscarriage were simply the absence of pregnancy and not an event in its own right. In this case pregnancy is figured even as a fortunate absence, a figment of gossip and story that can, consequently, disappear into the cheapest kind of general redemption.

3. See Grossberg 1997:353: "The act of power comes not in creating something from nothing, but in reducing something to nothing."

4. See Russo 1994 and, e.g., Chedgzoy 1995.

5. See Conquergood 1991; Phelan 1993.

6. See Foucault 1973.
7. See Butler 1990a on identity performance within a "heterosexual matrix."
8. See Walter Benjamin on the narrative costs of exiling death (1968:93–94):

> Dying was once a public process in the life of the individual and a most exemplary one; think of the medieval pictures in which the deathbed has turned into a throne toward which the people press through the wide-open doors of the death house. In the course of modern times dying has been pushed further and further out of the perceptual world of the living. There used to be no house, hardly a room, in which someone had not once died. . . . Today people live in rooms that have never been touched by death, dry dwellers of eternity, and when their end approaches they are stowed away in sanatoria or hospitals by their heirs. It is, however, characteristic that not only a man's knowledge or wisdom, but above all his real life—and this is the stuff that stories are made of—first assumes transmissible form at the moment of his death. Just as a sequence of images is set in motion inside a man as his life comes to an end—unfolding the views of himself under which he has encountered himself without being aware of it—suddenly in his expressions and looks the unforgettable emerges and imparts to everything that concerned him that authority which even the poorest wretch in dying possesses for the living around him. This authority is at the very source of the story.

9. Dr. Gustav Zinke, 1901, quoted in Leavitt 1986:177.
10. Medical intervention was and remains relatively routine for poor women, or for black women identified by race with class. Consumerism introduced a level of choice, echoed today in the trend toward "elective" inductions and cesarean sections.
11. Leavitt 1986:61, quoting William M. Gregory, 1912, in a letter to the editor of *JAMA* 58:577.
12. See Rich 1986, chapter 6, "Hands of Flesh, Hands of Iron."
13. See Leavitt 1986:117–140.
14. Note that recent innovations on external fetal monitoring will allow for increased mobility during labor.
15. *Right Start Catalogue* (Winter 1993:59).
16. The October 20, 1991, *Inforum* survey indicated that, if given a choice, 83 percent of women would choose an alternative to separate labor and delivery rooms but that only in 1991 did the number of women using these alternatives actually exceed the number in conventional arrangements. *Hospitals* 65:14.
17. According to the *Inforum* survey of October 20, 1991, despite the much publicized return of midwifery in the form of clinical nurse-midwives—again, an efficient choice for obstetric groups enabling them to maintain a large client pool at considerably reduced cost that also signified a potentially substantive

change in doctor-patient relations—only 7.4 percent of births in 1991 were reportedly attended by a "midwife or other."

18. I have relied on the methods of interviewing suggested by Slim and Thompson 1995; Camitta 1990; Gluck and Patai 1991; Langellier and Hall 1989; Oakley 1988; and Riessman 1987. On the insistence of the unversity review board, often against the wishes of the interviewees, all proper names have been changed to protect confidentiality; all interviews are quoted with written consent. Transcriptions have been minimally edited to account for performance values (tone, emphasis, pause, nonverbal behavior, etc.) and to correct for sense. The long-line verse style of transcription is, in general, intended to convey some sense of the rhythms of the speaking scene without the distractions of an elaborate symbol system transcription; see, e.g., Conquergood 1988; Deavere Smith 1993; Madison 1993; Fine 1984; and Tedlock's foundational work (1983). On the politics of transcription I have been particularly influenced by Frisch 1990.

19. See Martin 1987, chapter 11, "Class and Resistance." See also Ruth Behar's wonderful review of Martin (1990).

20. See Douglas 1966.

21. See Bhabha 1996 on the nature of a "partial" culture as opposed to more conventional conceptions of a culture as a bounded or, per Williams' classic formulation, "a whole way of life," and (1996:1–4) on the performative "imaginary of spatial distance" Bhabha variously characterizes as the " 'beyond' " and those " 'in-between' spaces" that "provide the terrain from elaborating strategies of selfhood—singular or communal—that initiate new signs of identity, and innovative sites of collaboration, and contestation, in the act of defining the idea of society itself"; see Phelan (1993:19) on performance as a mode of "active vanishing, a deliberate and conscious refusal to take the payoff of visibility."

22. On reflexive cultural critique, see Conquergood 1991; Strine 1991; as well as the long line of work on new ethnographic writing (including Tyler 1987 and Van Maanen 1988) for which Clifford and Marcus 1986 has become a landmark; and more recent innovations on feminist ethnography/oral history, e.g., Linden 1993; Visweswaran 1994; and Stewart 1996. On the prospects for a materialist "identity ethnography," see McRobbie 1992. On performance anthropology generally, see e.g., Turner 1986; Taussig 1987; Drewal 1992; and Schechner 1993; as well as Bell's useful critique (1992:37–54) of performance perspectives on ritual practice.

23. Related works are variously cited throughout the book but I want to recognize my basic debt to Langellier 1989 and Peterson and Langellier 1997 on the performance of women's everyday or "personal" narratives, and the interpretive example especially of Curti 1998; Madison 1998; Etter-Lewis and Foster 1996; Behar 1993; Madison 1993; and Riessman 1992, 1993, in the context of such work on the discourses of sexuality and maternity as Holland and Adkins 1996; Foster 1995; Case, Brett, and Foster 1995; Grosz and Probyn 1995; Mavor 1995;

Wiegman 1995; Butler 1994; Glenn, Chang, and Forcey 1994; Grosz 1994; Kibbey, Short, and Farmanfarmaian 1994; Kipnis 1993; Balsamo 1991; Kaplan 1992; Stanton 1992; Fuss 1991; Goldstein 1990; O'Barr, Pope, and Wyer 1990; Jaggar and Bordo 1989; Snitow, Stansell, and Thompson 1983.

24. There are many published accounts of birthing and maternity that importantly supplement textbook narratives. I am particularly grateful to Chesler 1979; Finger 1990; and Lazarre 1976 for their often daring ambivalence and critical perspectives. I am also intrigued by new opportunities to exchange birth stories over the Internet. I have not focused on print and digital forms of communication in this book, however, in favor of concentrating on the embodied act of telling and its particular prospects for hybridizing discourse.

25. See Bakhtin 1981. In this light I should also say that I feel cautioned by Allan Young when he poses, against the dangers of sentimentalizing, universalizing, or essentializing suffering and pain, the question "To what end are formations of suffering made?" (Young 1997).

26. See Sayre's definition (1989:25–26) of the performative artwork as the one that is undecidable vs. indeterminate, that "fans outward" in other performances and ongoing negotiations of possible meanings.

27. See Pollock 1998a; Phelan 1995; Modleski 1991:45–58; Mavor 1995; Nichols 1994:1–16; as well as Miller 1991 and Olson and Hirsh 1995.

28. See also Taussig 1992.

29. See Smith 1988 for a critical review of issues surrounding poststructural subjectivity. In general, I am relying on Hall's shift from issues of identity to identification, with the hope of contributing to a narrative politics that yields narrative formations *in the making*. See Hall 1996b.

30. I am responding here and throughout to Bertolt Brecht's sense of the loss of eros in the commodity marketplace. See Brecht 1971:376–378.

CHAPTER ONE: ORIGINS IN ABSENCE

1. See Diamond's elaboration (1996) of and corrective to Butler's prevailing version (1991) of performativity. For Diamond, the performative rule of *what's done* is always at risk of being undone in performance, in the corporeal collision of what's done with *doing* or in the act of *doing what's done*, in this case, telling myths of origin, repeating birth stories, representing ourselves in living genealogies (etymologies) of being.

2. Following Mikhail Bakhtin's sense of social identity formation as an ongoing, dialogic process, understanding dialogue as "not a means for revealing, for bringing to the surface the already ready-made character of a person" but as an unfinalizable process by which "a person . . . *becomes* for the first time that which he is." Bakhtin 1984:252.

3. Margaret, personal interview, May 28, 1992, hereafter quoted without further citation.

4. CVS, or chorionic villi sampling, is a prenatal genetic screening usually performed between the eighth and twelfth week of pregnancy. A recent innovation on amniocentesis, CVS promises early and quick results. And yet the risk of complications leading to miscarriage associated with CVS is approximately three in two hundred, three times higher than the rate associated with amniocentesis. The CVS procedure involves withdrawing chorionic villi—the fingerlike strands of genetic material projecting from the chorion or fetal membrane—through a long, thin catheter inserted into the uterus through the vagina.

5. Amniocentesis is a form of prenatal genetic testing usually performed between the sixteenth and eighteenth weeks of pregnancy, after sufficient amniotic fluid has accumulated and before abortion is no longer legally viable. It involves withdrawing a small amount of amniotic fluid (into which the developing fetus has shed cells) through a hollow needle inserted through the abdomen into the uterus. It is usually reserved for what are considered higher risk pregnancies.

6. Page duBois locates this notion of truth within an ancient tradition of torture as a means of discovery, by whose norms truth must be extracted from the body of the "other." See duBois 1991, especially 145–158.

7. Sonogram is the visual image of the fetus produced through the use of sound waves (sonography rather than X-ray) often referred to as "ultrasound." Sonography is generally used from the fifth week of pregnancy on to determine the condition of the fetus and the placenta, and to provide a visual guide for CVS and amniocentesis.

8. Laminaria are the seaweed strips inserted into the cervix to absorb uterine fluids in order to induce cervical ripening and dilatation. They are sometimes used in conjunction with external prostaglandin or intracervical gel.

9. In her critique of abstraction ("It doesn't *say* anything . . . it doesn't *do* anything") Margaret theorizes an alternative construction of knowledge, an epistemology drawing its strength not only from concrete experience but from its effectiveness and meaningfulness in context. In so doing, she favors not only the advice of her own body but embodied knowledge, knowledge that acts in and on the world, what Michael Eric Dyson calls the "performative epistemologies" characteristic of subaltern and popular cultures (Dyson 1993a). On the representation of "indigenous theory" in life narrative, see Madison 1998.

10. See Martha Nussbaum's critique (1986) of Agamemnon's tragic inference of rightness from necessity.

11. See Huet 1993 and Haraway 1992 on the reproduction of monstrosity.

12. Another interviewee, for instance, subjected first to a "loud, loud lecture" from her obstetrician and then to his stony, sulking silence, tells a story of playing him card for card. In her story she is the trickster who finally even makes his silence her virtue. "*I* never talked to *him!*" she insists, claiming his strategic withdrawal for her own tactical defense. Barbara and Jeff, personal interview, September 20, 1992.

13. Kathy and James, personal interview, May 23, 1992, hereafter cited without further citation.

14. Lila, personal interview, May 7, 1992, hereafter cited without further citation.

15. This image was suggested to me by Wagner 1994, per Braidotti 1991 and Butler 1990.

16. See de Lauretis 1984:119.

17. On the diversionary practice of "la perruque," especially as "a return of the ethical, of pleasure and of invention within the scientific institution," see de Certeau 1984.

18. Pitocin is generally administered through an IV drip (often one that is already supplying fluids and/or anesthetics to the birthing mother), hence Lila's references to taking the "pitocin drip."

19. See Eisenberg et al. 1984.

20. See e.g. Davis-Floyd 1992; Rothman 1991.

21. See also Kristeva 1982:4: "It is . . . not lack of cleanliness or health that cause abjection but what disturbs identity, system, order. What does not respect borders, positions, rules."

22. For a feminist deconstruction of the visible signs of pregnancy, see Martin 1990.

23. See Foucault's 1986 complementary claims for "heterotopias."

24. In thinking about Lila's love for Rosie, I can't help but recall Roland Barthes's sense of just how obsolete and so how transgressive the language of love has become. As Barthes says in his memoir: "Political liberation of sexuality: this is a double transgression, of politics by the sexual, and conversely. But this is nothing at all: let us now imagine reintroducing into the politico-sexual field thus discovered, recognized, traversed, and liberated . . . *a touch of sentimentality:* would that not be the *ultimate* transgression? the transgression of transgression itself? For, after all, that would be *love:* which would return: *but in another place*" (Barthes 1977:65–66).

25. The notion that maternity entails, following Freud, infantile regression, is even rehearsed at length in such a popular, trade book as Block 1990.

26. Kristeva most fully articulates the relation between the semiotic, *jouissance,* and the maternal body in "About Chinese Women," in which she is careful to note that *jouissance* is not identical with either ecstasy or madness but is constructed as such within the symbolic order it threatens: "It is thus that female specificity defines itself in patrilinear society: woman is a specialist in the unconscious, a witch, a baccanalian, taking her jouissance in an anti-Apollonian, Dionysian orgy" (Kristeva 1986a:154).

27. The notion of a "heterosexual matrix" substitutes in the work of some feminists for the reifications of oppression implicit in the repeated use of "patriarchy," e.g., Butler 1990.

28. Butler similarly argues against the Lacanian current in Kristeva that, she

claims, makes subversion "a futile gesture, entertained only in a derealized aesthetic mode which can never be translated into other cultural practices" (Butler 1990:78).

29. On libidinal economies of performance, see Bell 1995.

30. Rachel, personal interview, October 10, 1990.

CHAPTER TWO: NARRATIVE RITES

1. See Austin 1962, especially as qualified in Sedgwick 1993.

2. For fundamental articulations of play (following on the primary work of Bateson and Huizinga) with performance, see Turner 1982 and Conquergood 1989. Play takes on a particularly political significance in the postmodern context of, for instance, "ludic" feminism; see, e.g., Ebert 1996. Note also how contemporary theories of performativity describe the relay of identity through historical contingencies, especially per Butler 1990.

3. See Butler on gender (1990, 1993) as the sedimentation of performance in performativity; Conquergood's critique (1999) of the residual textualism in performance epistemologies; and Ricouer's early preference (1971) for texts as the sedimentation of meaning in time.

4. See, e.g., Fuss 1991:6–7: "Sexual identity may be less a function of knowledge than performance, or, in Foucauldian terms, less a matter of final discovery than perpetual reinvention." Fuss cites Butler 1990.

5. See Phelan 1993:13–27 for a complementary, Lacanian analysis of how the "ricochet" gaze produces an always already elusive self.

6. See, generally, Butler (1990, 1991, 1993) on the compulsory performance of sexed/gendered identities as well as Rich's primary discussion (1986b) of the ways in which heterosexuality is compelled.

7. This proposition is taken to its logical extreme in such recent neofictional works as Shields 1993 and Kincaid 1996 in which the authors/personae write their own births, performing their origins in the invention of auto/biography. For vigorously insightful, empirically based perspectives on the nature and value of self-narration, see Myerhoff 1978, 1982.

8. As Probyn 1993:2 has argued of the self generally.

9. Probyn's recent work (1996) on identity becoming or "becoming-other" as it is articulated through desire, traversal, and belonging is extraordinarily provocative in this regard. I am particularly indebted to her cautionary sense that "working within positivity does not necessarily result in a celebratory rhetoric; rather, desire as a social force compels us to think beyond the terminal points of either celebration or *ressentiment*. I write in order to remind myself of the ways in which belonging hinges on not-belonging, to raise the ways in which the manners of being at the threshold may provide another perspective from which to view the complexities of identity, difference, subjectivity, and desire." Probyn 1996:14. See also Brown 1995.

10. See Forte's characterization (1992) of "erotic agency," per Diamond 1996:4. See also Diamond's useful distinction (1996:4–5) between the "doing" and the "done" in performative acts: "Gender . . . is both a doing—a performance that puts conventional gender attributes into possibly disruptive play—and a thing done—a pre-existing oppressive category." Diamond importantly identifies "doing" and "done" as simultaneous dimensions of any given performative act, which nonetheless suggests the practical conundrum of "doing what's done," i.e., raising the possibility that the play implicit in "doing" may be curtailed in the repetition of normative behaviors, even assimilated to the legitimation of those norms by repetition and/or the possibility that the transitive, embodied (carnival? parodic?) act of performance might break through the (re)citational chains of performativity.

11. See Trinh 1989:136 on the erotics of oral historical transmission. I am indebted here to Cixous 1976 and Suleiman 1990, as well as to Hebdige's sense (1988:242) that "the seat of being is the belly. . . . We shall have to learn again that the belly is the vital organ: the mother of the world, the medieval seat of the humours, the organ of the appetites, digestion and laughter."

12. Note de Certeau's sense that "the story's first function is to authorize, or more exactly, to *found*," which, for de Certeau has the spatial implication of "creating a theater of actions" (1984:123).

13. In general, assuming Bakhtin's fundamental principles of dialogue and polyphony (1981, 1984).

14. For an alternative, autobiographical account of maternal abjection, see, e.g., Allison 1992, 1996, especially per Allison's wish (1996:46) to "demythologize" poverty.

15. Anticipating Butler 1993:4 on the performative politics of disidentification: "Although the political discourses that mobilize identity categories tend to cultivate identifications in the service of a political goal, it may be that the persistence of disidentification is equally crucial to the rearticulation of democratic contestations. Indeed, it may be precisely through practices which underscore disidentification with those regulatory norms by which sexual differance is materialized that both feminist and queer politics are mobilized. Such collective disidentification can facilitate a reconceptualization of which bodies matter, and which bodies are yet to emerge as critical matters of concern."

16. On the possibilities of performing "beyond reproduction" compare with Phelan on the prospects for representation without reproduction (1993:3): "The pleasure of resemblance and repetition produces both psychic assurance and political fetishization. Representation reproduces the Other as the Same. Performance, insofar as it can be defined as representation without reproduction, can be seen as a model for another representational economy, one in which the reproduction of the Other as the Same is not assured."

17. Rachel and John, personal interview, October 8, 1990, hereafter quoted without further citation.

18. See Huet 1993 on the authority of resemblance in narratives of "monstrous" maternity. Note too that Annie's miraculous arrival was matched and doubled three years later by the birth of her brother, David. David was also born by in vitro fertilization but with spina bifida, one of the most complicated congenital birth disorders, which in his case meant that a small hole at the base of his spine exposed the spinal cord's trailing nerve ends. After corrective surgery, adding miracle to miracle, David quickly and completely recovered.

19. See Russo 1994 on feminist aspects of the spectacular grotesque.

20. See Bakhtin 1984, especially pp. 48–49, on the regenerative potential of the grotesque. Bakhtin specifically evokes the proximity of life/death in the space of "carnival truth" where, he argues, "the world is destroyed so that it may be regenerated and renewed. While dying it gives birth." He elaborates: "The grotesque liberates man from all the forms of inhuman necessity that direct the prevailing concept of the world. This concept is uncrowned by the grotesque and reduced to the relative and the limited. Necessity, in every concept which prevails at any time, is always one-piece, serious, unconditional, and indisputable. But historically the idea of necessity is relative and variable. The principle of laughter and the carnival spirit on which the grotesque is based destroys this limited seriousness and all pretense of an extratemporal meaning and unconditional value of necessity. It frees human consciousness, thought, and imagination for new potentialities."

21. Hebdige is drawing generally on Bakhtin 1984b.

22. See Schrager 1983 on "progressive structuring of detail" in oral history. See Madison 1999 on performance as the "performance of possibilities."

23. Similarly, Russo imagines (1994:167, 171) substituting "aerial surveillance" for the panoptical gaze through the figure of the female aerialist.

24. See also Schechner 1988:xiii on what he takes to be one of the premiere principles of performance: "Sometimes . . . it is necessary to live as if 'as if' = 'is.' "

25. For a summary of performative challenges to conventional approaches to historiography, see Pollock 1998b. See also Blocker 1999 and Hall 1998.

26. I am fundamentally indebted to Turner 1982, 1986 and Bauman 1977, 1986 for my sense of the operative dynamics of performance in everyday life and to Dwight Conquergood, for introducing me to both.

27. See, in general, Foucault 1979, 1978, 1970.

28. See Fiske 1993:90 on the visceral significance of these events: "These peak experiences matter so intensely because they integrate identity with the body: they are ones of significance rather than signification. And their significance matters so much that they often serve as nodal points around which other experiences are organized."

29. See Stone 1988 on family stories generally.

30. See, e.g., Fuss's 1991 analysis of the "inside/out" construction of difference.

31. See Russo's important qualification (1994:64–65) of Bakhtin's identification of the maternal body with the "grotesque" body.

32. For a more elaborate analysis of the performance of gynecological exams, see Kapsalis 1997.
33. See, e.g., Russo 1994; Rowe 1995.
34. See also Taussig 1980.
35. See Martin 1987 on the discourses of menstruation as waste.
36. For an especially incisive account of the Foucauldian "origins" and effects of reproductive technologies, especially insofar as they produce new subjects (fit mothers, unfit mothers, infertile women), see Sawicki 1991. See also Diamond and Quinby 1988. Farquhar 1996 locates IVF within broader discourses of reproductive technologies. For general critique of reproductive technologies as social apparati and the position of women within scientific discourses, see Adams 1994; Duden 1993; Franklin 1992; Hartouni 1991; Jacobus, Keller, and Shuttleworth 1990; Petchesky 1987; Rothman 1989; Treichler, Cartwright, and Penley 1998. For excellent critical overviews of emerging and ambivalent relationships between feminist theory and the rise of repro-tech, see Charlesworth 1995 and Caddick 1995. See Seltzer 1992 for a useful history of the mechanization of gendered bodies.
37. See Lugones 1987 on "world"-traveling as a strategic means of "loving perception."
38. Note that for Bakhtin (1981:360) the "hybrid is not only double-voiced and double-accented . . . but is also double-languaged; for in it there are not only . . . two individual consciousnesses, two voices, two accents, as there are two sociolinguistic consciousnesses, two epochs" that are not unconsciously mixed but that "come together and consciously fight it out on the territory of the utterance." Where hybridity has remained unconscious, however, it has also been "at the same time profoundly productive historically." Unconscious hybrids "are pregnant with potential for new world views, with new 'internal forms' for perceiving the world in words." Hence, Bhabha (1996:58) claims the kind of hybridity Rachel performs for resistance: "Strategies of hybridization reveal an estranging movement in the 'authoritative,' even authoritarian inscription of the cultural sign. At the point at which the precept attempts to objectify itself as a generalized knowledge or a normalizing, hegemonic practice, the hybrid strategy or discourse opens up a space of negotiation where power is unequal but its articulation may be equivocal. Such negotiation . . . makes possible the emergence of an 'interstitial' agency that refuses the binary representation of social antagonism. Hybrid agencies find their voice in a dialectic that does not seek cultural supremacy or sovereignty. They deploy the partial culture from which they emerge to construct visions of community, and versions of historic memory, that give narrative form to the minority positions they occupy."
39. See Turner's discussion (1982:120–121) of the dialectics of performing "not-not-me," borrowing on Schechner, Brecht, and Winnecott.
40. See, e.g., Homi Bhabha on performative duplicities (1990:3).

CHAPTER THREE: PRACTICING PAIN

As I indicate in chapter 1, I am attracted to Kristeva's sense of language and maternity but withdraw from some of the more explicitly psychoanalytic dimensions and implications of her work. Here, as in chapter 1, I use and rely on Kristeva selectively.

1. See, for instance, the McGill-Melzack Pain Questionnaire, which initiated a more "experiential" approach to pain by providing patients with an adjectival base for naming pain but remained taxonomic in its assortment of two to five descriptors per each of twenty categories keyed, as David Morris observes, to white middle-class "experience." See Morris 1991:16–17.

2. I am grateful to Judith Farquhar for suggesting this point.

3. See Morris 1991:35.

4. See, e.g., duBois 1991.

5. Following Scheper-Hughes and Lock 1987 and, e.g., Sacks 1985.

6. The image of the shadow is drawn from Leavitt 1986:13–35, " 'Under the Shadow of Maternity.' "

7. See Morris 1991:9–30: "Living Pain: Mystery or Puzzle?"

8. Karen, personal interview, June 5, 1992; hereafter quoted without further citation.

9. I am using *entangled* in Susan Suleiman's sense, through Lacan, of the relationship between the narrator, Jacques Hold, and the title character, Lol V. Stein, in Marguerite Duras's novel, *The Ravishing of Lol V. Stein* , which Suleiman describes as that of a "subject to subject, not subject to object." In this particularly performative relation, Jacques and Lol are reciprocally "ravished." See Suleiman 1990:112–118.

10. I remain skeptical of the extent to which a "woman's culture" built on tacitness, as a kind of secret fetish world—especially when it is cast as a "separate sphere"—may confirm the kind of gendered normativity implicit in, for instance, Luce Irigaray's apparently utopic question "How, within this society, can women initiate certain rites that allow them to live and become women in all dimensions? How are systems of exchange to be set *among women?*" (Irigaray 1993b:80). I'd like to suggest here, as throughout this volume, that instead of constituting a closed economy "*among women*" birth stories circulate as forms or currency of maternal as well as carnival and dialectical (per Scott 1990) power.

11. Kristeva 1986b:167.

12. Borrowing on Simone de Beauvoir's (1952) classic formulation.

13. Alicia Ostriker 1986 would argue, moreover, that this is the impulse behind much of the feminine/feminist poetics from the mid-seventies. Thanks to T. J. Snyder for introducing me to the LeGuin story.

14. See, e.g., Edelman 1992 on American anxieties about anality. Note also the correlation of Karen's narrative body to the distinction Bakhtin 1984b draws between the open, rent, seeping "grotesque" body and the sealed "classical" body.

15. Borrowing on Foucault 1977.
16. In an everyday, prototypical form of Boal's 1979 "rehearsal for the revolution" (thanks to Jodi Kanter for pointing this out). See also Boal 1995 and Cohen-Cruz and Schutzman 1994, as well as Bowman's useful review (1995) of the latter.
17. Karen also used the former WIC (Women, Infants, and Children) program.
18. AFDC: Aid to Families with Dependent Children; personal communication, December 1995.
19. Seremetakis 1991:4 cites Morinis 1985; Scarry 1985; Taussig 1987.
20. Seremetakis 1991:4–5 cites Comaroff 1985 and Taussig 1987 as primary examples. Drawing especially on Lakoff 1987 and Abu Lughod 1986, she describes emotions as "embodied, conceptual, moral, and ideational constructs that place the self in a dynamic relation to social structure." See also Cvetkovich 1992 on the politics of affect in the context of rising industrialization and the emergence of "mass culture."
21. See Martin, Gutman, and Hulton 1988.
22. Andrea, personal interview, July 18, 1991; hereafter quoted without further citation.
23. See also Morris's complementary discussion (1991:118–124), per Kristeva, of "psychic numbing" in the novels of Marguerite Duras, and Russo's critique (1994:64) of Kristeva's description of the "abject" maternal body.
24. See Alcoff 1991.
25. Regarding the emerging genre of illness narratives, see, among others, Kleinman 1988 and Frank 1995. See also Mairs's lively critique (1994) of "The Literature of Personal Disaster."
26. During the seventh month of my second pregnancy I had an appointment with one of the two female obstetricians in a private practice. Falsely assuming that a woman—by virtue of being a woman—would be receptive, I broached the idea of a birth plan. I began by explaining that the speed of my first birth made me concerned that I wouldn't have time to specify preferences or to make effective decisions during the second, knowing that second births are typically shorter than first births, often by as much as half. She immediately recoiled, claiming birth plans "make me feel resentful" and asking, "What, you think I don't know my business?" She backed up to assure me that every case was unique, that there were no "routines," and that doctors have incorporated much of what midwives do. When I asked about routine fetal monitoring, she went on to say, "No no no—unless of course there's meconium in the waters—and, oh yes, we do routinely break the waters; of course if you don't want the monitor, we can have you sign all kinds of release forms and you can do whatever you want." I left the office feeling abandoned to an ultimatum: either I yield total control or I risk alienating my support staff and take complete responsibility for whatever happens. Angry and anxious, a part of me nonetheless also felt triumphant for having discerned the contradictions in her posi-

tion—the gap between her explicit denial of routine and the fact that a myriad of procedures were apparently so routine as to be unrecognizable as such. Beneath the anger and pleasure was, however, a deeper disappointment in not being able to expect anything from her based on the biological status of our shared "femaleness." Could some of the same disappointment be informing these stories? For a counterperspective on women healers, see Perrone, Stockel, Krueger 1989.

27. See Russo 1994. On the logics of the medical/anatomical gaze, see, e.g., Cartwright 1995; and Foucault 1994, especially chapter 7, "Seeing and Knowing," and chapter 9, "The Visible Invisible."

28. See also Sullivan 1989 and, more generally, Samuel and Thompson 1990.

29. Janet, interview conducted by Elyse, June 21, 1991.

30. Rachel, personal interview, October 8, 1990.

31. Denise, personal interview, January 22, 1992.

32. Yvonne, personal interview, June 1, 1993.

33. Janet, personal interview conducted by Elyse, June 21, 1991

34. Elyse, personal interview, May 14, 1991.

35. Saundra, personal interview, June 23, 1992.

36. Janet, personal interview conducted by Elyse, June 21, 1991.

37. Sue, personal interview, November 1, 1991.

38. Charlotte, personal interview, May 2, 1991.

39. Deborah, personal interview, August 13, 1992.

40. I am indebted to Jacquelyn Hall for raising these questions.

41. See Morris 1991:37–40.

42. Freud has perhaps most notably imagined female desire through Dora, whose apparent incoherence marks her/it, for Freud, "hysterical." Subsequent feminists, especially French theorists of *l'écriture féminine*, have reclaimed the open, disruptive, excessive desire pathologized in Freud to narratives of female/feminine subversion. See Freud 1963 and, e.g., Irigaray 1993b:164–165; Suleiman 1990; and Barthes 1975. On the fundamental principles of *l'écriture féminine*, especially as it relates to a maternal order, see Cixous 1976; and Irigaray 1993a:59: "What this implies is that the female body is not to remain the object of men's discourse or their various arts but that it become the object of a female subjectivity experiencing and identifying itself."

43. On the genealogy of experience, see Scott 1991 and Roach 1996.

44. Re: cultural "contact zones," see Conquergood 1991.

CHAPTER FOUR: SECRETS/DOUBLES

1. See, e.g., Spacks 1985.

2. Phelan cites Butler (1990:106): "The confusion between the real and the representational occurs because 'the real is positioned both before and after its representation; and representation becomes a moment of the reproduction and

consolidation of the real.' " See Phelan's general critique of visibility politics, especially chapter 6, "White Men and Pregnancy: Discovering the Body to Be Rescued," and its conclusion: "Often the one who never appears is the one running the show" (Phelan 1993:145).

3. See duBois 1991, especially chapter 14, "Women, the Body, and Torture," pp. 145–158.

4. My sense of what constitutes local knowledge certainly derives from Geertz 1983 but depends more specifically on Fiske's sense (1993) of how "localizing" practices resist dominant knowledge formations and Haraway's critical distinction (1991) between conversational and discovery modes of knowledge. On histories of opposition to what has variously been called shamming, theatricality, and performance, see Barish 1981. For an important corrective to the categories of "sincerity" and "authenticity" on which such opposition is in part founded, see Bowman 1998.

5. See Scott 1990:3.

6. See Conquergood 1998.

7. Re: the talk show especially in relation to Foucault's critique (1978) of confessional discourses, see Alcoff and Gray 1993 and Shattuc 1997, and, from an informed but, I think, more sentimental perspective, Plummer 1995:97–112. On the hyper-real (Baudrillard 1983) effects of the talk show phenomenon, see also White 1992 and Nichols 1994, especially chapter 3, "At the Limits of Reality (TV)."

8. See, e.g., Madison 1998; Etter-Lewis and Foster 1996; Battaglia 1995.

9. On how sexual stories are compelled and distorted by particular narrative frameworks, see Alcoff and Gray 1993 and my own reflections on performing sexual harassment, Pollock 1994.

10. While I am trying to suggest the performative power of secrecy, I recognize that telling secrets, under some conditions, may indeed be powerful. See, for instance, Schneider's discussion (1996) of the performance artist, Annie Sprinkle, reknowned for turning the female body "inside out" in performances that invite audience members to view her cervix. The performance demystifies the exoticization of female interiority. It moreover, as Schneider argues, turns the "eye" at the center of this secret back on the spectator, who otherwise performs specular/speculum control: seeing the cervix, he/she is seen—and the hierarchies of specular control are at least temporarily suspended in the reciprocities of being looked at.

11. Jaylin, personal interview, December 6, 1990.

12. Randy and Doug, personal interview, February 11, 1991.

13. Elyse's "new moms" group, personal interview, conducted by Elyse, June 21, 1991.

14. See Scott 1990 on the dialectics of "hidden" and official transcripts.

15. See Debord's foundational work (1977) on commodification by spectacle; and Roach 1996, especially on marketing black bodies.

16. Note how Feldman (1991:12) negotiated the "domain of secret knowledge" in Northern Ireland:

    In a culture of political surveillance, participant observation is at best an absurdity and at least a form of complicity with those outsiders who surveil. I avoided residing in the communities of my informants for these reasons. Neutral spaces were best for talking about the items we agreed to deal with. Long-term visual appropriation of any social milieu was not welcomed. Too much mobility between adversarial spaces, which my nationality facilitated, also proved to be subjectively disturbing. As I became familiar with the topography of confessional communities, I realized that only other people who were moving back and forth in such a manner were the police and the army. I had to constrain the body as well as the voice. Finally, in order to know I had to become expert in demonstrating that there were things, places, and people I did not want to know.

    Feldman projects an ethic of dialogic "spacing." See also Modell 1988 on how an interviewer may be compelled to positions of advocacy and support or written into the interviewees' script for performance.

17. "Hiding in the open": to be distinguished from Hebdige's use (1988) of "hiding in the light" to describe youth culture's translation of surveillance into the pleasures of being watched.
18. Quoted with the permission of the author.
19. Ruth, personal interview, June 26, 1996, hereafter quoted without further citation.
20. In this way Ruth took up Donna Haraway's sense (1991:201) of the world as Coyote, the trickster figure prominent in Native American legends, the "witty actor and agent" of transformation, "the coding trickster with whom," Haraway insists, "we must learn to converse." See Conqergood's 1999 elaboration.
21. See Sedgwick 1993a.
22. For a vigorous elaboration and critique of Fanon, see Pellegrini 1997, especially chapter 5, "Through the Looking Glass: Fanon's Double Vision." On the dialectics of "other" identification, see also Fuss 1991, especially her incisive introduction.
23. As opposed, for instance, to the kind of colonial mimicry Bhabha 1984 describes. Note also Fanon (1967:116): even under conditions of radical overdetermination, "everything takes on a new guise."
24. See also Dyson (1993b:67–69) on the ethical implications of subverting "common perceptions of the culturally or physically possible through the creative and deceptive manipulation of appearance."
25. Compare with Bourdieu's primary category (1977:76) of "the habitus" as "a socially constituted system of cognitive and motivating structures."
26. With all the "seriousness" Victor Turner (1982) attributes to play.

27. I am indebted here to Cohen and Dhiambo 1998.

28. For more broadly historical critique of raced identity, reproduction, and class, see Lawson and Rhode 1993 and Solinger 1992.

29. Sedgwick 1993 has argued that "unknowing" (in the form, for example, of Americans' refusal to learn other languages or an employer's claim not to know that AIDS isn't infectious on contact) can hold global and sexual politics to conservative, white, middle-class agendae. In this light, it could be that the interviewer is frustrated not only by Ruth's presumed secrecy but by her appropriation of a middle-class privilege—or her suspicion, latent or otherwise, that she has been caught out in her own strategic ignorance.

30. See hooks 1992, "The Oppositional Gaze," on the translation of being looked at into looking, as well as her return interrogation, "Representations of Whiteness."

31. See Fuss 1991.

32. See Butler 1990 on how identity is sedimented in performativity. For Butler, the trick of performativity—that nonetheless signifies possibilities for subversion—lies in the extent to which it hides itself from itself, in the extent to which it consolidates the *appearance* of a natural or given identity through repetition. See also Gilroy, " ' . . . to be real': The Dissident Forms of Black Expressive Culture," and hooks, "Performance Practice as a Site of Opposition," in Ugwu 1995.

33. See Stabile 1992 as well as Phelan's sense (1993:145) that "in place of the [Lacanian] split subject and the drama of lack, the pregnant woman raises the spectacle of a double-subject and the drama of overwhelming presence."

34. See Cixous 1986 on the identification of woman with nature within a broadscale series of masculinist dichotomies; see also Cixous 1976 for her feminist reversion of the same, especially as developed in Suleiman 1990:179–180, "The Laugh of the Mother." See Bakhtin's distinction (1984b) between the "grotesque" and "classical" body, elaborated in Stallybrass and White 1986.

35. I am using *masquerade* loosely here, although I am borrowing on Riviere's sense of femininity (1986) as a masquerade or a performative compensation for a lack; accordingly, the secret of masquerade is that there is no secret, that there is *nothing there* that is not constituted in performance.

36. Compare with Pellegrini 1997:97 on what she calls "racial gateways": "entry points through which members of socially subordinated and racialized groups might pass over to the other side." For Pellegrini, the gateway is a figure for passing, for gaining privilege by, e.g., mastering the language of privileged groups. I want to suggest that insofar as racial gateways are points of passing over by passing *for*—with all of the social and psychic difficulties, even terror, passing implies (see Larsen 1986; Ginsberg 1996)—they are also points of leakage and permeation, of passing in and out, and hence particularly dense and contested points of identity formation.

37. For the recent history of homebirthing in the United States, see O'Connor 1993.
38. Information obtained in informal conversations as well as from the *Raleigh News and Observer,* May 12, 1991, and December 5, 1994. I am particularly grateful to Smith and Holmes 1996 and Ulrich 1990 on the history of lay midwifery.
39. Ellen, personal interview, August 7, 1992, hereafter quoted without further citation.
40. Reflecting Turner's sense (1969) that the liminal phase of ritual refreshes pre/antistructural principles of social relation.
41. As opposed to, for instance, what Phelan calls (1993:3) the "pleasure of resemblance and repetition."
42. My use of *liminal* here derives specifically from Victor Turner's emphasis on the primary stage of ritual and social, redressive dramas, which he has defined in a number of contexts, including his essay (1986:41) on the anthropology of experience, which seems most relevant here:

> The *limen*, or threshold, a term I borrowed from van Gennep's second of three stages in rites of passage, is a no-man's-land betwixt and between the structural past and the structural future as anticipated by the society's normative control of biological developments. It is ritualized in many ways, but very often symbols expressive of ambiguous identity are found cross culturally: androgynes, theriomorphic figures, monstrous combinations of elements drawn from nature and culture, with some symbols such as caverns, representing both birth and death, womb and tomb. I sometimes talk about the liminal phase being dominantly in the subjunctive mood of culture, the mood of maybe, might be, as if, hypothesis, fantasy, conjecture, desire. . . . Ordinary life is in the indicative mood, where we expect the invariant operation of cause and effect, of rationality and commonsense. Liminality can perhaps be described as a fructile chaos, a storehouse of possibilities, not a random assemblage but a striving after new forms and structures, a gestation process, a fetation of modes appropriate to postliminal existence.

See also Turner 1982, 1984.
43. Charlotte, personal interview, May 2, 1991, hereafter quoted without further citation.
44. See Treichler 1990 on the implications of birth understood as a "double medical emergency." See also Treichler 1989.
45. See Phelan 1991 on performative reckonings; Pollock 1998b on the problems and possibilities of history as disappearance. I am grateful to Berlant 1996 for characterizing memory as invention vs. mourning and the refusal to reproduce.

46. Suggested by Dyson's characterization (1993b:67) of the "will to spontaneity" in African-American culture(s) as "the way in which historical accidence is transformed into cultural advantage, and the way acts of apparently random occurrence are spontaneously and imaginatively employed by Africans and African-Americans in a variety of forms of cultural expression," in conversation with Tony Perucci, June 1997.

47. Connie Conant, "Every Purpose Under Heaven": unpublished poem, quoted with permission of the author. I am grateful to Connie for talking with me and sharing poems of her daughter's stillbirth.

48. This perspective is meant to complement compelling and vital arguments for what Anzaldúa calls "overcoming the tradition of silence" (1990) and what Bell and Apfel 1995, drawing on Haraway 1991, for instance, describe as the power gained by changing the relationship between the "seer and the seen" in contexts of visibility. I also want to recognize, with hooks (1989, 1990), that where we think we see silence may be powerful, longstanding traditions of speech and story.

49. Echoing Foucault's qualification (1994:115) of what he takes to be the basic postulate of medical perception: "that all that is *visible* is *expressible*, and that it is *wholly visible* because it is *wholly expressible*": "Total description is a present and ever-withdrawing horizon; it is much more the dream of a thought than a basic conceptual structure."

50. Whether characterized by the domestic(ating) name of "mystery" or, e.g., "abjection" (Kristeva 1982), the "uncanny" (Freud; see Russo 1994), the "originary dark" (Sedgwick), the "unspeakable" (Tyler 1987). I cannot help but think of Jane Blocker's beautiful work (1999) on Ana Mendieta in this regard.

51. Including even the recent spate of highly publicized teenage "neonaticides" and "hidden" pregnancies. See coverage in *Newsweek*, July 7, 1997. Compare with Scheper-Hughes 1992 on infanticide in Brazil.

52. See Chesler (1979:101): "I have no one to talk to about this. Women's smiles are fixed grins: the grimace of masks, of silence. I know they smell my fear, want not to remember their own. They keep their distance."

53. As Roach claims (1996:25), citing Foucault (1977:142) in his compelling argument for performance genealogies: "What is and is not 'behind things' [is] not the timeless and essential secret, but the secret that they have no essence or that their essence was fabricated in a piecemeal fashion from alien forms. . . . What is found at the historical beginning of things is not the inviolable identity of their origin; it is the dissension of other things. It is disparity."

54. See Bourdieu 1977 on the fundamental concept of "symbolic capital."

55. Suggested by Lauren Berlant 1996, referring to Morrison 1993, 1970. Note also Morrison (1990:305) on the importance of "emotional memory—what the nerves and the skin remember as well as how it appeared."

56. Suggested by Hebdige 1988:231, quoting Deleuze and Guattari 1983. Compare with Seremetakis 1991 on rural Greek mourning practices. Seremetakis (1991:14) asks:

> What perspectives emerge if, as opposed to observing death through the lens of social structure, or culture/nature, we examine these categories through the optic of death? In other words, can theory shift from the familiarization of death to the defamiliarization of the social order by death?

Abu Lughod, Lila. 1986. *Veiled Sentiments: Honor and Poetry in a Bedouin Society.* Berkeley: University of California Press.

Adams, Alice E. 1994. *Reproducing the Womb: Images of Childbirth in Science, Feminist Theory, and Literature.* Ithaca: Cornell University Press.

Alcoff, Linda. 1991. "The Problem of Speaking for Others." *Cultural Critique* 20:5–32.

Alcoff, Linda and Laura Gray. 1993. "Survivor Discourse: Transgression or Recuperation?" *Signs: Journal of Women in Culture and Society* 18.2:260–290.

Allison, Dorothy. 1996. "A Question of Class." In Linny Stovall, ed., *Secrets.* Hillsboro, Ore.: Blue Heron.

— 1992. *Bastard Out of Carolina.* New York: Penguin.

Anzaldúa, Gloria. 1987. *Borderlands/La Frontera: The New Mestiza.* San Francisco: Aunt Lute.

Austin, J. L. 1962. *How to Do Things with Words.* Cambridge: Harvard University Press.

Bakhtin, M. M. 1984a. *Problems of Dostoevsky's Poetics.* Ed. and trans. Caryl Emerson. Minneapolis: University of Minnesota Press.

— 1984b. *Rabelais and His World.* Trans. Helene Iswolsky. Bloomington: Indiana University Press.

— 1981. *The Dialogic Imagination.* Ed. Michael Holquist, trans. Caryl Emerson and Michael Holquist. Austin: University of Texas Press.

Balsamo, Anne. 1991. Feminism and Cultural Studies. *Journal of Midwest MLA* 24:50–73.

Barish, Jonas. 1981. *The Anti-Theatrical Prejudice* . Berkeley: University of California Press.

Barker, Francis. 1984. *The Tremulous Private Body: Essays on Subjection*. New York: Methuen.

Barthes, Roland. 1977. *Roland Barthes by Roland Barthes*. Trans. Richard Howard. New York: Noonday.

— 1975. *The Pleasure of the Text*. New York: Hill and Wang.

Battaglia, Deborah, ed. 1995. *Rhetorics of Self-Making*. Berkeley: University of California Press.

Baudrillard, Jean. 1983. *Simulations*. New York: Semiotext(e).

Bauer, Dale M. and S. Jaret McKinstry, eds. 1991. *Feminism, Bakhtin, and the Dialogic*. Albany: State University of New York Press.

Bauman, Richard. 1986. *Story, Performance, and Event: Contextual Studies of Oral Narrative*. New York: Cambridge University Press.

— 1977. *Verbal Art as Performance*. Prospect Heights, Ill.: Waveland.

Behar, Ruth 1993. *The Translated Woman: Crossing the Border with Esperanza's Story*. Boston: Beacon.

— 1990. "The Body in the Woman, the Story in the Woman: A Book Review and Personal Essay." In Laurence Goldstein, ed., *The Female Body. Michigan Quarterly Review* (special issue) 29.4:695–738.

Bell, Catherine. 1992. *Ritual Theory, Ritual Practice*. New York: Oxford University Press.

Bell, Elizabeth. 1995. "Toward a Pleasure-Centered Economy: Wondering a Feminist Aesthetics of Performance." *Text and Performance Quarterly* 15.2:99–121.

Bell, Susan and Roberta J. Apfel. 1995. "Looking at Bodies: Insights and Inquiries about DES-Related Cancer." *Qualitative Sociology* 18.1:3–20.

Benjamin, Walter. 1968. *Illuminations*. New York: Schocken.

Berlant, Lauren. 1996. "Remembering Love, Forgetting Everything Else: Now Voyager." Public lecture, October 25, 1996, University of North Carolina at Chapel Hill.

Bhabha, Homi K. 1996. "Culture's In-Between." In Stuart Hall and Paul du Gay, eds., *Questions of Cultural Identity*, pp. 53–60. Thousand Oaks, Cal.: Sage.

— 1994. *The Location of Culture*. New York: Routledge.

— 1990. "Introduction: Narrating the Nation." In Homi Bhabha, ed., *Nation and Narration*, pp. 1–7. New York: Routledge.

— 1984. "Of Mimicry and Man: The Ambivalence of Colonial Discourse." *October* 28:125–133.

Binchy, Maeve. 1990. *Circle of Friends*. New York: Dell.

Block, Joyce. 1990. *Motherhood as Metamorphosis*. New York: Penguin.

Blocker, Jane. 1999. *Where is Ana Mendieta? Identity, Performativity, and Exile*. Durham: Duke University Press.

Boal, Augusto. 1995. *The Rainbow of Desire: The Boal Method of Theater and Therapy*. Trans. Adrain Jackson. New York: Routledge.

— 1979. *The Theater of the Oppressed*. Trans. Charles A. McBride and Maria-Odilia Leal McBride. New York: Theater Communications Group.

Bourdieu, Pierre. 1977. *Outline of a Theory of Practice*. Trans. Richard Nice. New York: Cambridge University Press.

Bowman, Ruth. 1998. "Performing Social Rubbish: Humbug and Romance in the American Marketplace." In Della Pollock, ed., *Exceptional Spaces: Essays in Performance and History*, pp. 121–141. Chapel Hill: University of North Carolina Press.

— 1995 (1994). "Playing Boal: Theater, Therapy, Activism." Review. In *Text and Performance Quarterly* 15.3:255–256.

Braidotti, Rosi. 1991. *Patterns of Dissonance: A Study of Women in Contemporary Philosophy*. New York: Routledge.

Brecht, Bertolt. 1971. "Preface to *Drums in the Night*." In Ralph Mannheim and John Willett, eds., *Collected Plays*, 1:376–377. New York: Vintage.

Brown, Wendy. 1995. "Wounded Attachments: Late Modern Oppositional Political Formations." In John Rajchman, ed., *The Identity in Question*, pp. 200–227. New York: Routledge.

Butler, Judith. 1994. *More Gender Trouble: Feminism Meets Queer Theory. differences* (special issue) 6.

— 1993. *Bodies That Matter: On the Discursive Limits of "Sex."* New York: Routledge.

— 1990a. *Gender Trouble: Feminism and the Subversion of Identity*. New York: Routledge.

— 1990b. "The Force of Fantasy: Feminism, Mapplethorpe, and Discursive Excess." *differences* 2.2:105–125.

Caddick, Alison. 1995. "Making Babies, Making Sense: Reproductive Technologies, Postmodernity, and the Ambiguities of Feminism." In Paul A. Komesaroff, ed., *Troubled Bodies: Critical Perspectives on Postmodernism, Medical Ethics, and the Body*, pp. 142–167. Durham: Duke University Press.

Camitta, Miriam. 1990. "Gender and Method in Folklore Fieldwork." *Southern Folklore* 47.2:21–32.

Carpenter, Carole. 1985. "Tales Women Tell: The Function of Birth Experience Narratives." *Canadian Folklore* 47.1/2:21–34.

Cartwright, Lisa. 1995. "Gender Artifacts: Technologies of Bodily Display in Medical Culture." In Lynne Cooke and Peter Wollen, eds., *Visual Display*, pp. 218–235. Seattle: Bay.

Case, Sue Ellen, Philip Brett, and Sue Leigh Foster, eds. 1995. *Cruising the Performative: Interventions Into the Representation of Ethnicity, Nationality, and Sexuality*. Bloomington, Indiana: Indiana University Press.

Charlesworth, Max. 1995. "Whose Body? Feminist Views on Reproductive Technologies." In Paul A. Komesaroff, ed., *Troubled Bodies: Critical Perspectives on*

Postmodernism, Medical Ethics, and the Body, pp. 125–141. Durham: Duke University Press.

Chedgzoy, Kate. 1995. "Frida Kahlo's Grotesque Bodies." In Penny Florence and Dee Reynolds, eds., *Feminist Subjects, Multi-Media: Cultural Methodologies*, pp. 39–57. New York: Manchester University Press.

Chesler, Phyllis. 1979. *With Child: A Diary of Motherhood*. New York: Crowell.

Chodorow, Nancy. 1978. *The Reproduction of Mothering: Psychoanalysis and the Sociology of Gender*. Berkeley: University of California Press.

Cixous, Hélène. 1986. "Sorties." *The Newly Born Woman*, pp. 63–134. Trans. Betsy Wing. Minneapolis: University of Minnesota Press.

— 1976. "The Laugh of the Medusa." Trans. Keith Cohen and Paula Cohen. *Signs: Journal of Women and Culture in Society* 1.4:875–893.

Clifford, James and George E. Marcus, eds. 1986. *Writing Culture: The Poetics and Politics of Ethnography*. Berkeley: University of California Press.

Cohen, David William and E. S. Atieno Odhiambo. 1998. "Reading the Minister's Remains: Investigations into The Death of The Honourable Minister John Robert Ouko in Kenya, February, 1990." In Della Pollock, ed., *Exceptional Spaces: Essays in Performance and History*, pp. 77–97. Chapel Hill: University of North Carolina Press.

Cohen-Cruz, Jan and Mady Schutzman, eds. 1994. *Playing Boal: Theatre, Therapy, Activism*. New York: Routledge.

Comaroff, Jean. 1985. *Body of Power, Spirit of Resistance: The Culture and History of a South African People*. Chicago: University of Chicago Press.

Conquergood, Dwight. 1999. "Beyond the Text: Toward a Performative Cultural Politics." In Sheron Dailey, ed., *The Future of Performance Studies*. Washington D.C.: National Communication Association.

— 1993. "Storied Worlds and the Work of Teaching." In *Communication Education* 42.4:337–348.

— 1991. "Rethinking Ethnography: Toward a Critical Cultural Poetics." *Communication Monographs* 58:179–194.

— 1989. "Poetics, Play, Process, and Power: The Performative Turn in Anthropology." *Text and Performance Quarterly* 9.1:82–88.

— 1988. "Health Theater in a Hmong Refugee Camp: Performance, Communication, and Culture." *TDR: The Drama Review* 32.3: 174–208.

Curti, Lidia. 1998. *Female Stories, Female Bodies: Narrative, Identity, and Representation*. New York: New York University Press.

Cvetkovich, Ann. 1992. *Mixed Feelings: Feminism, Mass Culture, and Victorian Sensationalism*. New Brunswick, N.J.: Rutgers University Press.

Davis-Floyd, Robbie. 1992. *Birth as an American Rite of Passage*. Berkeley: University of California Press.

Deavere Smith, Anna. 1993. *Fires in the Mirror*. New York: Doubleday.

de Beauvoir, Simone. 1952. *The Second Sex*. Trans. H. M. Parshley. New York: Knopf.

Debord, Guy. 1977. *Society of the Spectacle*. Detroit: Black and Red.

de Certeau, Michel. 1984. *The Practice of Everyday Life*. Trans. S. Rendall. Berkeley: University of California Press.

de Lauretis, Teresa. 1984. "Desire in Narrative." In Teresa de Lauretis, *Alice Doesn't*, pp. 103–157. Bloomington: Indiana University Press.

Deleuze, Gilles and Felix Guattari. 1983. *On the Line*. Trans. John Johnston. New York: Semiotext(e).

Diamond, Elin, ed. 1996. *Performance and Cultural Politics*. New York: Routledge.

Diamond, Irene and Lee Quinby, eds. 1988. *Feminism and Foucault: Reflections on Resistance*. Boston: Northeastern University Press.

Douglas, Mary. 1966. *Purity and Danger: An Analysis of Concepts of Pollution and Taboo*. New York: Praeger.

Drewal, Margaret Thompson. 1992. *Yoruba Ritual: Performers, Play, Agency*. Bloomington: Indiana University Press.

duBois, Page. 1991. *Torture and Truth*. New York: Routledge.

Duden, Barbara. 1993. *Disembodying Women: Perspectives on Pregnancy and the Unborn*. Cambridge, Massachusetts: Harvard University Press.

Dyson, Michael Eric. 1993a. Public lecture, December 1993, University of North Carolina at Chapel Hill.

—. 1993b. *Reflecting Black: African-American Cultural Criticism*. Minneapolis: University of Minnesota Press.

Ebert, Teresa L. 1996. *Ludic Feminism and After: Postmodernism, Desire, and Labor in Late Capitalism*. Ann Arbor: University of Michigan Press.

Edelman, Lee. 1992. "Tearooms and Sympathy; or, The Epistemology of the Water Closet." In Andrew Parker, Mary Russo, Doris Summer, and Patricia Yeager, eds., *Nationalisms and Sexualities*, pp. 263–284. New York: Routledge.

Eisenberg, Arlene, Heidi Eisenberg Murkoff, and Sandee Eisenberg Hathaway, eds. 1984. *What to Expect When You're Expecting*. New York: Workman.

Etter-Lewis, Gwendolyn and Michele Foster, eds. 1996. *Unrelated Kin: Race and Gender in Women's Personal Narratives*. New York: Routledge.

Fanon, Frantz. 1967. *Black Skin, White Masks*. Trans. Charles Lam Markmann. New York: Grove.

Farquhar, Dion. 1996. *The Other Machine: Discourse and Reproductive Technologies*. New York: Routledge.

Feldman, Allen. 1991. *Formations of Violence: The Narrative of the Body and Political Terror in Northern Ireland*. Chicago: University of Chicago Press.

Fernandez, James W. 1986. *Persuasions and Performances: The Play of Tropes in Culture*. Bloomington: Indiana University Press.

Fetterly, Judith. 1978. *The Resisting Reader*. Bloomington: Indiana University Press.

Fine, Elizabeth C. 1984. *The Folklore Text: From Performance to Print*. Bloomington: Indiana University Press.

Finger, Anne. 1990. *Past Due: A Story of Disability, Pregnancy, and Birth*. Seattle: Seal.

Fiske, John. 1993. *Power Plays, Power Works*. New York: Verso.

Forte, Jeannie. 1992. "Focus on the Body: Pain, Praxis, and Pleasure in Feminist Performance." In Joseph Roach and Janelle Reinelt, eds., *Critical Theory and Performance*, pp. 248–262. Ann Arbor: University of Michigan Press.

Foster, Susan. 1995. *Corporealities*. New York: Routledge.

Foucault, Michel. 1994. *The Birth of the Clinic: An Archaeology of Medical Perception*. Trans. A. M. Sheridan Smith. New York: Vintage.

— 1986. "Of Other Spaces." *Diacritics* (Spring): 22–27.

— 1979. *Discipline and Punish: The Birth of the Prison*. Trans. Alan Sheridan. New York: Pantheon.

— 1978. *The History of Sexuality*. Vol. 1: *An Introduction*. Trans. Robert Hurley. New York: Vintage.

— 1977. "Nietzsche, Genealogy, History." In Donald F. Bouchard, ed., *Language, Counter-Memory, Practice*, pp. 139–164. Trans. Donald F. Bouchard and Sherry Simon. Ithaca: Cornell University Press.

— 1973. *The Birth of the Clinic: An Archaeology of Medical Perception*. Trans. A. M. Sheridan Smith. New York: Vintage.

— 1970. *The Order of Things: An Archaeology of the Human Sciences*. London: Tavistock.

Frank, Arthur. 1995. *The Wounded Storyteller: Body, Illness, and Ethics*. Chicago: University of Chicago Press.

Franklin, Sarah. 1992. "Fetal Fascinations: New Dimensions to the Medical-Scientific Construction of Fetal Personhood." In Sarah Franklin, Celia Lury, and Jackie Stacey, eds., *Off-Center: Feminism and Cultural Studies*, pp. 190–205. New York: Harper-Collins.

Freud, Sigmund. 1963. *Dora: An Analysis of a Case of Hysteria*. Ed. Philip Rieff. New York: Macmillan.

Frisch, Michael. 1990. *A Shared Authority: Essays on the Craft and Meaning of Oral and Public History*. Albany: State University of New York Press.

Fuss, Diana, ed. 1991. *Inside/Out: Lesbian Theories, Gay Theories*. New York: Routledge.

Geertz, Clifford. 1983. *Local Knowledge*. New York: Basic.

Gibson, Pamela Church and Roma Gibson, eds. 1993. *Dirty Looks: Women, Pornography, Power* . London: BFI.

Ginsberg, Elaine K., ed. 1996. *Passing and the Fictions of Identity*. Durham: Duke University Press.

Glenn, Evelyn Nakano, Grace Chang, and Linda Rennie Forcey, eds., 1994. *Mothering: Ideology, Experience, and Agency*. New York: Routledge.

Gluck, Sherna Berger and Daphne Patai, eds. 1991. *Women's Words: The Feminist Practice of Oral History*. New York: Routledge.

Goldstein, Laurence, ed. 1990, 1991. *The Female Body. Michigan Quarterly Review* (special issues) 29.4, 30.1.

Grossberg, Lawrence. 1997. *Bringing It All Back Home: Essays on Cultural Studies.* Durham: Duke University Press.

Grosz, Elizabeth. 1994. *Volatile Bodies: Toward a Corporeal Feminism.* Bloomington: Indiana University Press.

Grosz, Elizabeth and Elspeth Probyn, eds. 1995. *Sexy Bodies: The Strange Carnalities of Feminism.* New York: Routledge.

Hall, Jacquelyn. 1998. "You Must Remember This: Autobiography as Social Critique." *Journal of American History* (September 1998): 439–465.

Hall, Stuart. 1996a. "The After-Life of Frantz Fanon: Why Fanon? Why Now? Why *Black Skin, White Masks?*" Public lecture, April 15, University of North Carolina at Chapel Hill.

— 1996b. Introduction. In Stuart Hall and Paul du Gay, eds., *Questions of Cultural Identity*, pp. 1–17. London: Sage.

Haraway, Donna. 1992. "The Promise of Monsters: A Regenerative Politics for Inappropriate/d Others." In Lawrence Grossberg, Cary Nelson, and Paula Treichler, eds., *Cultural Studies*, pp. 295–337. New York: Routledge.

— 1991. "Situated Knowledges: The Science Question and the Privilege of Partial Perspective." In Donna Haraway, *Simians, Cyborgs, and Women: The Reinvention of Nature*, pp. 183–201. New York: Routledge.

Hartouni, Valerie. 1991. "Containing Women: Reproductive Discourse in the 1980s." In Constance Penley and Andrew Ross, eds., *Technoculture*, pp. 27–56. Minneapolis: University of Minnesota Press.

Hebdige, Dick. 1988. *Hiding in the Light.* New York: Routledge.

Hirsch, Marianne. 1989. *The Mother/Daughter Plot: Narrative, Psychoanalysis, Feminism.* Bloomington: Indiana University Press.

Hitchcock, Peter. 1993. *Dialogics of the Oppressed.* Minneapolis: University of Minnesota Press.

Holland, Janet and Lisa Adkins, eds. 1996. *Sex, Sensibility, and the Gendered Body.* New York: St. Martin's.

hooks, bell. 1992. *Black Looks: Race and Representation.* Boston: South End.

— 1990. "Homeplace: A Site of Resistance." In bell hooks, *Yearning*, pp. 41–49. Boston: South End.

— 1989. *Talking Back: Thinking Feminist, Thinking Black.* Boston: South End.

Huet, Marie-Hélène. 1993. *Monstrous Imagination.* Cambridge: Harvard University Press.

— 1982. *Rehearsing the Revolution: The Staging of Marat's Death.* Berkeley: University of California Press.

Irigiray, Luce. 1993a. *Je, Tu, Nous: Toward a Culture of Difference.* Trans. Alison Martin. New York: Routledge.

— 1993b. *Sexes and Genealogies.* Trans. Gillian C. Gill. New York: Columbia University Press.

— 1991. "This Sex Which Is Not One." In Robyn R. Warhol and Diane Price Herndl, eds., *Feminisms*, pp. 350–356. New York: Routledge.

— 1980. "When Our Lips Speak Together." *Signs: Journal of Women and Culture in Society* 6.11:69–79.

Jackson, Michael. 1989. *Paths Toward a Clearing: Radical Empiricism and Ethnographic Inquiry*. Bloomington: Indiana University Press.

Jacobus, Mary, Evelyn Fox Keller, and Sally Shuttleworth, eds. 1990. *Body/Politics: Women and the Discourses of Silence*. New York: Routledge.

Jaggar, Alison M. and Susan R. Bordo, eds. 1989. *Gender/Body/Knowledge: Feminist Reconstructions of Being and Knowing*. New Brunswick, New Jersey: Rutgers University Press.

Jordan, Brigitte, 1993. *Birth in Four Cultures: A Crosscultural Investigation of Childbirth in Yucatan, Holland, Sweden, and the United States*. 4th. ed. Prospect Heights, Ill.: Waveland.

Kaplan, E. Ann. 1992. *Motherhood and Representation: The Mother in Popular Culture and Melodrama*. New York: Routledge.

Kapsalis, Terri. 1997. *Public Privates*. Durham: Duke University Press.

Kibbey, Ann, Kayann Short, and Abouali Farmanfarmaian, eds. 1994. *Sexual Artifice: Persons, Images, Politics*. New York: New York University Press.

Kincaid, Jamaica. 1996. *The Autobiography of My Mother*. New York: Farrar Straus Giroux.

Kipnis, Laura. 1993. *Ecstasy Unlimited: On Sex, Capital, Gender, and Aesthetics*. Minneapolis: University of Minneapolis Press.

Kleinman, Arthur. 1988. *The Illness Narratives: Suffering, Healing, and the Human Condition*. New York: Basic.

Kristeva, Julia. 1986a. "About Chinese Women." In Toril Moi, ed., *The Kristeva Reader*, pp. 138–159. New York: Columbia University Press.

— 1986b. "Stabat Mater." In Toril Moi, ed., *The Kristeva Reader*, pp. 160–186. Oxford: Blackwell.

— 1982. *Powers of Horror: An Essay on Abjection*. New York: Columbia University Press.

— 1980. "Motherhood According to Bellini." In Julia Kristeva, *Desire in Language: A Semiotic Approach to Literature and Art*, pp. 237–270. New York: Columbia University Press.

Lakoff, George. 1987. *Women, Fire, and Dangerous Things*. Chicago: University of Chicago Press.

Lakoff, George and Mark Johnson. 1980. *Metaphors We Live By*. Chicago: University of Chicago Press.

Langellier, Kristin and Deanna Hall. 1989. "Interviewing Women: A Phenomenological Approach to Feminist Communication Research." In Kathryn Carter and Carole Spitzack, eds., *Doing Research on Women's Communication*, pp. 193–220. Norwood, N.J.: Ablex.

Larsen, Nella. 1986. *Quicksand* and *Passing*. Ed. Deborah McDowell. New Brunswick, N.J.: Rutgers University Press.

Lawson, Annette and Deborah C. Rhode, eds. 1993. *The Politics of Pregnancy: Adolescent Sexuality and Public Policy.* New Haven: Yale University Press.

Lazarre, Jane. 1986. *The Mother Knot.* Boston: Beacon.

Leavitt, Judith Walzer. 1986. *Brought to Bed: Childbearing in America, 1750–1950* New York: Oxford University Press.

Lefebvre, Henri. 1987. "The Everyday and Everydayness." Trans. Christine Levich, with Alice Kaplan and Kristin Ross. *Yale French Studies* 73:7–11.

LeGuin, Ursula. 1985. "She Unnames Them." *New Yorker* (January 21): 27.

Linden, Ruth. 1993. *Making Stories, Making Selves: Feminist Reflections on the Holocaust.* Columbus: Ohio State University Press.

Lugones, Maria. 1994 (1987). "Playfulness, 'World'-Travelling, and Loving Perception." In D. Soyini Madison, ed., *The Woman That I Am: The Literature and Culture of Contemporary Women of Color,* pp. 626–637. New York: St. Martin's.

McRobbie, Angela. 1992. "Post-Marxism and Cultural Studies: A Post-Script." In Lawrence Grossberg, Cary Nelson, and Paula Treichler, eds., *Cultural Studies,* pp. 719–730. New York: Routledge.

Madison, D. Soyini. 1999. "Performance, Personal Narratives, and the Politics of Possibility." In Sheron Dailey, ed., *The Future of Performance Studies.* Washington, D.C.: National Communication Association.

— 1998 (1993). " 'That Was My Occupation': Oral Narrative, Performance, and Black Feminist Thought." In Della Pollock, ed., *Exceptional Spaces: Essays in Performance and History,* pp. 319–342. Chapel Hill: University of North Carolina Press.

Mairs, Nancy. 1996. *Carnal Acts.* Boston: Beacon.

— 1995, 1989. *Remembering the Bone House: An Erotics of Place and Space.* Boston: Beacon.

— 1994. *Voice Lessons: On Becoming a (Woman) Writer.* Boston: Beacon.

Martin, Emily. 1987. *The Woman in the Body: A Cultural Analysis of Reproduction.* Boston: Beacon.

Martin, Joanne. 1990. "Deconstructing Organizational Taboos: The Suppression of Gender Conflict in Organizations." *Organization Science* 1.4:339–59.

Martin, Luther, Huck Gutman, and Patrick H. Hulton. 1988. *Technologies of the Self: A Seminar with Michel Foucault.* Amherst: University of Massachusetts Press.

Mavor, Carol. 1995. *Pleasures Taken: Performances of Sexuality and Loss in Victorian Photographs.* Durham: Duke University Press.

Michaelson, Karen, ed. 1988. *Childbirth in America: Anthropological Perspectives.* South Hadley, Mass.: Bergin and Garvey.

Miller, D. A. 1988. *The Novel and the Police.* Berkeley: University of California Press.

Modell, Judith. 1988. "The Performance of Talk: Interviewing Birthparents and Adoptees." *International Journal of Oral History* 9.1:6–26.

Modleski, Tania. 1991. *Feminism Without Women: Culture and Criticism in a "Post-feminist" Age*. New York: Routledge.

Morinis, Alan. 1985. "The Ritual Experience: Pain and the Transformation of Consciousness in Ordeals of Initiation." *Ethos* 13.2:150–175.

Morris, David B. 1991. *The Culture of Pain*. Berkeley: University of California Press.

Morrison, Toni. 1993 (1970). "Afterword." In Toni Morrison, *The Bluest Eye*, pp. 209–216. New York: Plume.

— 1990. "The Site of Memory." In Russell Ferguson, Martha Gever, Trinh T. Minh-ha, Cornel West, eds., *Out There: Marginalization and Contemporary Cultures*, pp. 299–305. Cambridge: MIT Press.

— 1987. *Beloved*. New York: Plume.

Myerhoff, Barbara. 1982. "Telling One's Story." *Center Magazine* 8.2:22–40.

— 1978. *Number Our Days*. New York: Simon and Schuster.

Nichols, Bill. 1994. *Blurred Boundaries: Questions of Meaning in Contemporary Culture*. Bloomington: Indiana University Press.

Norton, Catherine Sullivan. 1989. *Life Metaphors: Stories of Ordinary Survival*. Carbondale: Southern Illinois University Press.

Nussbaum, Martha. 1986. *The Fragility of Goodness: Luck and Ethics in Greek Tragedy and Philosophy*. New York: Cambridge University Press.

O'Barr, Jean, Deborah Pope, and Mary Wyer, eds. 1990. *Ties That Bind: Essays on Mothering and Patriarchy*. Chicago: University of Chicago Press.

O'Connor, Bobbie B. 1993. "The Home Birth Movement in the United States." *Journal of Medicine and Philosophy* 18.2:147–174.

Oakley, Ann. 1988. "Interviewing Women." In Helen Roberts, ed., *Doing Feminist Research*, pp. 30–61. Boston: Routledge and Kegan Paul.

Olson, Gary A. and Elizabeth Hirsh. 1995. *Women Writing Culture*. Albany: State University of New York.

Ostriker, Alicia. 1986. *Stealing the Language: The Emergence of Women's Poetry in America*. Boston: Beacon.

Pellegrini, Ann. 1997. *Performance Anxieties: Staging Psychoanalysis, Staging Race*. New York: Routledge.

Petchesky, Rosalind. 1987. "Foetal Images: The Power of Visual Culture in the Politics of Reproduction." In Michelle Stanworth, ed., *Reproductive Technologies: Gender, Motherhood, and Medicine*, pp. 57–80. Minneapolis: University of Minnesota Press.

Peterson, Eric E. 1987. "The Stories of Pregnancy: On Interpretation of Small Group Cultures." *Communication Quarterly* 35.1:39–47.

Peterson, Eric E. and Kristin M. Langellier. 1997. "The Politics of Personal Narrative Methodology." *Text and Performance Quarterly* 17.2:135–152.

Phelan, Peggy. 1995. "Thirteen Ways of Looking at Choreographing Writing." In Susan Foster, ed., *Choreographing History*, pp. 200–210. Bloomington: Indiana University Press.

— 1993. *Unmarked: The Politics of Performance.* New York: Routledge.

Plummer, Ken. 1995. *Telling Sexual Stories: Power, Change, and Social Worlds.* New York: Routledge.

Pollock, Della. 1998a. "Performing Writing." In Peggy Phelan and Jill Lane, eds., *The Ends of Performance.* New York: New York University Press.

— 1998b. "Introduction: Making History Go." In Della Pollock, ed., *Exceptional Spaces: Essays in Performance and History.* Chapel Hill: University of North Carolina Press

— 1994. "(Un)Becoming Voices: Representing Sexual Harassment in Performance." In Shereen Bingham, ed., *Conceptualizing Sexual Harassment as Discourse,* pp. 107–126. Westport, Conn.: Praeger.

Probyn, Elspeth. 1996. *Outside Belongings.* New York: Routledge.

— 1993. *Sexing the Self: Gendered Positions in Cultural Studies.* New York: Routledge.

Rich, Adrienne. 1986a (1976). *Of Woman Born: Motherhood as Experience and Institution.* New York: Norton.

— 1986b (1980). "Compulsory Heterosexuality and Lesbian Existence." In Adrienne Rich, *Blood, Bread, and Poetry: Selected Prose, 1979–1985,* pp. 631–660. New York: Norton.

Ricouer, Paul. 1971. "The Model of the Text: Meaningful Action Considered as a Text." *Social Research* 38:529–562.

Riessman, Catherine Kohler. 1993. *Narrative Analysis.* Newbury Park, Cal.: Sage.

— 1992. "Making Sense of Marital Violence: One Woman's Narrative." In George C. Rosenwald and Richard L. Ochberg, eds., *Storied Lives: The Cultural Politics of Self-Understanding,* pp. 231–249. New Haven: Yale University Press.

— 1987. "When Gender Is Not Enough: Women Interviewing Women." *Gender and Society* 1:172–207.

Riviere, Joan. 1986. "Womanliness as Masquerade." In Victor Burgin, James Donald, and Cora Kaplan, eds., *Formations of Fantasy,* pp. 35–44. New York: Methuen.

Roach, Joseph. 1996. *Cities of the Dead: Circum-Atlantic Performance.* New York: Columbia University Press.

Rothman, Barbara Katz. 1991. *In Labor: Women and Power in the Birthplace.* New York: Norton.

— 1989. *Recreating Motherhood: Ideology and Technology in a Patriarchal Society.* New York: Norton.

Rowe, Kathleen. 1995. *The Unruly Woman: Gender and the Genres of Laughter.* Austin: University of Texas Press.

Ruddick, Sara. 1989. *Maternal Thinking: Toward a Politics of Peace.* New York: Ballantine.

Russo, Mary. 1994. *The Female Grotesque: Risk, Excess, and Modernity.* New York: Routledge.

Sacks, Oliver. 1985. *Migraine: Understanding a Common Disorder.* Berkeley: University of California Press.

Samuel, Raphael and Paul Thompson. 1990. *The Myths We Live By.* New York: Routledge.

Sayre, Henry M. 1989. *The Object of Performance: The American Avant-Garde Since 1970.* Chicago: University of Chicago Press.

Scarry, Elaine. 1985. *The Body in Pain: The Making and Unmaking of the World.* New York: Oxford University Press.

Schechner, Richard. 1993. *The Future of Ritual.* New York: Routledge.

— 1988. *Performance Theory.* New York: Routledge.

Schely-Newman, Esther. 1995. "Sweeter Than Honey: Discourse of Reproduction Among North-African Israeli Women." *Text and Performance Quarterly* 15.3:175–188.

Scheper-Hughes, Nancy. 1992. *Death Without Weeping: The Violence of Everyday Life in Brazil.* Berkeley: University of California Press.

Scheper-Hughes, Nancy and Margaret Lock. 1987. "The Mindful Body: A Prolegomenon to Future Work in Medical Anthropology." *Medical Anthropology Quarterly* 1:6–39.

Schrager, Samuel. 1983. "What is Social in Oral History?" *International Journal of Oral History* 4.2:76–98.

Scott, James. 1990. *Domination and the Arts of Resistance: Hidden Transcripts.* New Haven: Yale University Press.

Scott, Joan. 1991. "The Evidence of Experience." *Critical Inquiry* 17.4:773–797.

Sedgwick, Eve Kosofsky. 1993a. "Privilege of Unknowing: Diderot's *The Nun.*" In Eve Kosofsky Sedgwick, *Tendencies,* pp. 23–51. Durham: Duke University Press.

— 1993b. "Queer Performativity: Henry James's *The Art of the Novel.*" *Gay and Lesbian Quarterly* 1.1:1–16.

— 1990. "Introduction: Axiomatic." In Eve Kosofsky Sedgwick, *Epistemology of the Closet,* pp. 1–63. Berkeley: University of California Press.

Sellers, Susan, ed. 1994. *The Hélène Cixous Reader.* New York: Routledge.

Seltzer, Mark. 1992. *Bodies and Machines.* New York: Routledge.

Seremetakis, C. Nadia. 1991. *The Last Word: Women, Death, and Divination in Inner Mani.* Chicago: University of Chicago Press.

Shattuc, Jane M. 1997. *The Talking Cure: TV Talk Shows and Women.* New York: Routledge.

Shields, Carol. 1993. *The Stone Diaries.* New York: Penguin.

Slim, Hugo and Paul Thompson. 1995. *Listening for a Change: Oral Testimony and Community Development.* Philadelphia: New Society.

Smith, Margaret Charles and Linda Janet Holmes. 1996. *Listen to Me Good: The Life Story of an Alabama Midwife.* Columbus: Ohio State University Press.

Smith, Paul. 1988. *Discerning the Subject.* Minneapolis: University of Minnesota Press.

Snitow, Ann, Christine Stansell, and Sharon Thompson, eds. 1983. *Powers of Desire: The Politics of Sexuality.* New York: Monthly Review.

Solinger, Rickie. 1992. *Wake Up Little Susie: Single Pregnancy and Race Before Roe v. Wade*. New York: Routledge.

Spacks, Patricia Meyer. 1985. *Gossip*. Chicago: University of Chicago Press.

Stabile, Carol. 1998 (1992). "Shooting the Mother: Fetal Photography and the Politics of Disappearance." In Paula A. Treichler, Lisa Cartwright, and Constance Penley, eds., *The Visible Woman: Imaging Technologies, Gender, and Science*, pp. 171–197. New York: New York University Press.

Stallybrass, Peter and Allon White. 1986. *The Politics and Poetics of Transgression*. Ithaca: Cornell University Press.

Stanton, Donna C., ed. 1992. *Discourses of Sexuality: From Aristotle to AIDS*. Ann Arbor: University of Michigan Press.

Steedman, Carolyn Kay. 1986. *Landscape for a Good Woman: A Story of Two Lives*. New Brunswick, N.J.: Rutgers University Press.

Stewart, Kathleen. 1996. *A Space on the Side of the Road: Cultural Poetics in an "Other" America*. Princeton: Princeton University Press.

Stone, Elizabeth. 1988. *Black Sheep and Kissing Cousins: How Our Family Stories Shape Us*. New York: Times.

Strine, Mary S. 1991. "Critical Theory and 'Organic' Intellectuals: Reframing the Work of Cultural Critique." *Communication Monographs* 58:195–201.

Suleiman, Susan Rubin. 1990. *Subversive Intent: Gender, Politics and the Avant-Garde*. Cambridge, Massachusetts: Harvard University Press.

Taussig, Michael. 1992. *The Nervous System*. New York: Routledge.

— 1987. *Shamanism, Colonialism, and the Wild Man: A Study in Terror and Healing*. Chicago: University of Chicago Press.

— 1980. Reification and the Consciousness of the Patient. *Social Science and Medicine* 14:3–13.

Tavris, Carol. 1992. *The Mismeasure of Woman*. New York: Simon and Schuster.

Tedlock, Dennis. 1983. *The Spoken Word and the Work of Interpretation*. Philadelphia: University of Pennsylvania Press.

Treichler, Paula. 1990. "Feminism, Medicine, and the Meaning of Childbirth." In Mary Jacobus, Evelyn Fox Keller, and Sally Shuttleworth, eds., *Body/Politics Women and the Discourses of Science*, pp. 113–138. New York: Routledge.

— 1989. "What Definitions Do: Childbirth, Cultural Crisis, and the Challenge to Medical Discourse." In Brenda Dervin, Lawrence Grossberg, Barbara J. O'Keefe, and Ellen Wartella, eds., *Rethinking Communication*. Vol. 2: *Paradigm Exemplars*, 2:424–453. Thousand Oaks, Cal.: Sage.

Treichler, Paula A., Lisa Cartwright, and Constance Penley, eds., 1998. *The Visible Woman: Imaging Technologies, Gender, and Science*. New York: New York University Press.

Turner, Victor W. 1986a. *The Anthropology of Performance*. New York: Performing Arts Journal.

— 1986b. "Dewey, Dilthey, and Drama: An Essay in the Anthropology of Experience." In Victor W. Turner and Edward M. Bruner, eds., *The Anthropology of Experience*, pp. 33–44. Urbana: University of Illinois Press.

—— 1984. "Liminality and the Performative Genres." In John J. MacAloon, ed., *Rite, Drama, Festival, Spectacle: Rehearsals Toward a Theory of Cultural Performance*, pp. 19–41. Philadelphia: Institute for the Study of Human Issues.

—— 1982. *From Ritual to Theater: The Human Seriousness of Play*. New York: Performing Arts Journal.

Tyler, Stephen. 1987. *The Unspeakable: Discourse, Dialogue, and Rhetoric in the Postmodern World*. Madison: University of Wisconsin Press.

Ugwu, Catherine, ed. 1995. *Let's Get It On: The Politics of Black Performance*. Seattle: Bay.

Ulrich, Laurel Thatcher. 1990. *A Midwife's Tale*. New York: Knopf.

Umansky, Lauri. 1996. *Motherhood Reconceived: Feminism and the Legacy of the Sixties*. New York: New York University Press.

Van Maanen, John. 1988. *Tales of the Field: On Writing Ethnography*. Chicago: University of Chicago Press.

Visweswaran, Kamala. 1994. *Fictions of Feminist Ethnography*. Minneapolis: University of Minnesota Press.

Wagner, Andrea Townsend. 1994. "Narrating Bodies: The Play of Sexuality and Gender in an Interview Scene." M.A. thesis, University of North Carolina, Chapel Hill.

Ward, Frazer. 1992. "Foreign and Familiar Bodies." In Jesús Fuenmayor, Kate Haug, and Frazer Ward, *Dirt and Domesticity: Constructions of the Feminine*, pp. 8–37. New York: Whitney Museum of American Art.

White, Mimi. 1992. *Tele-Advising: Therapeutic Discourse in American Television*. Chapel Hill: University of North Carolina, Chapel Hill.

Wiegman, Robyn. 1995. *American Anatomies: Theorizing Race and Gender*. Durham: Duke University Press.

Young, Allan. 1997. "Twins, Birds, and Atrocities: An Episode in the Recent History of Traumatic Memory." Public lecture, January 23, University of North Carolina at Chapel Hill.